Skin Grafts for Successful Wound Closure

Edited by Madhuri Gore

Published in London, United Kingdom

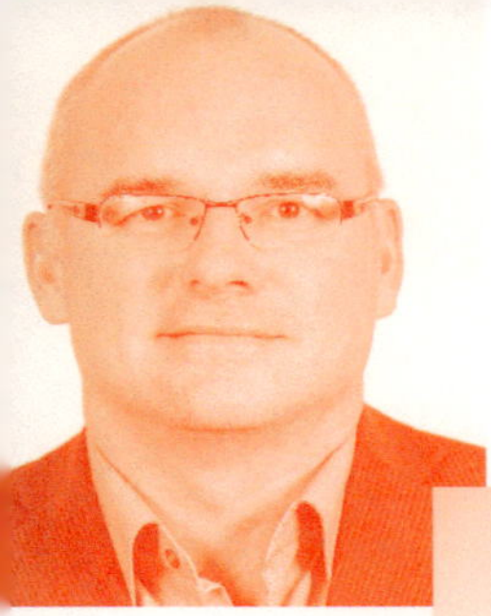
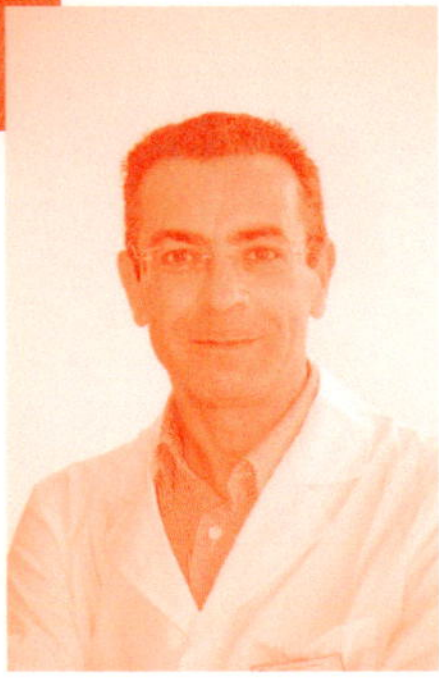
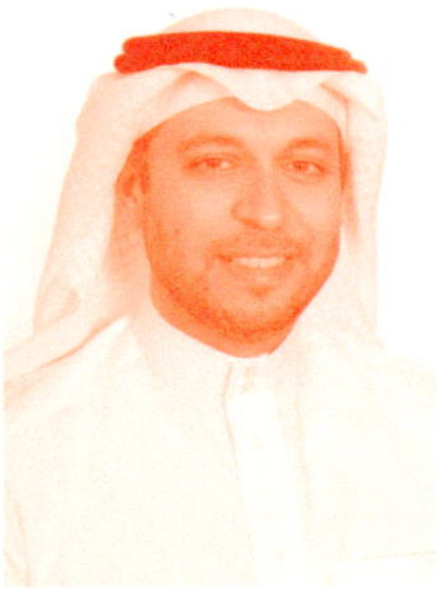
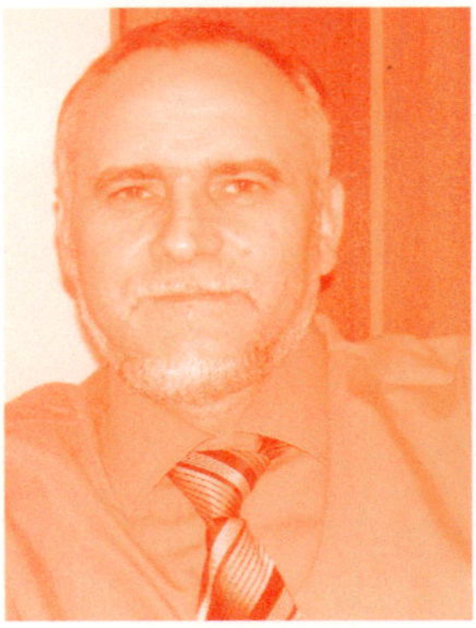
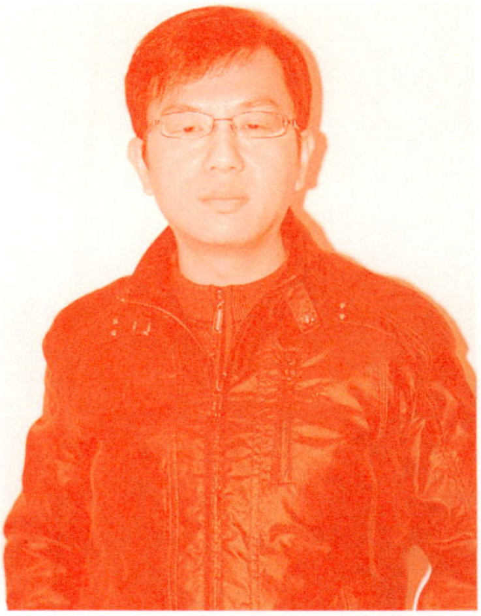
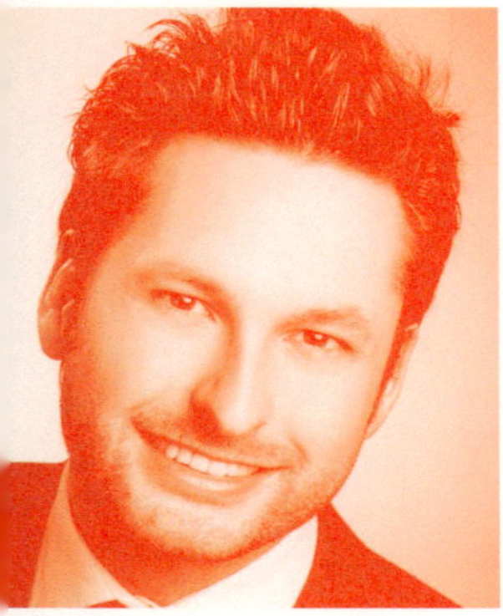
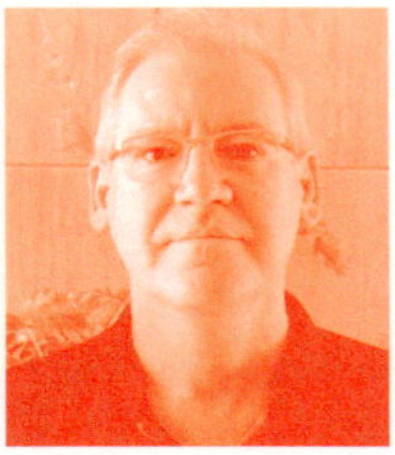

IntechOpen

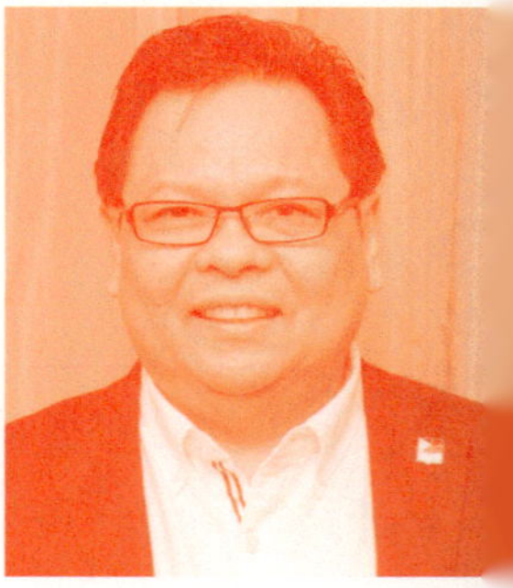
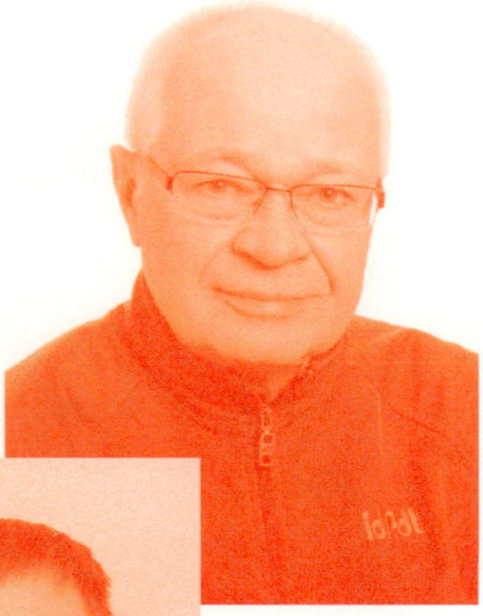
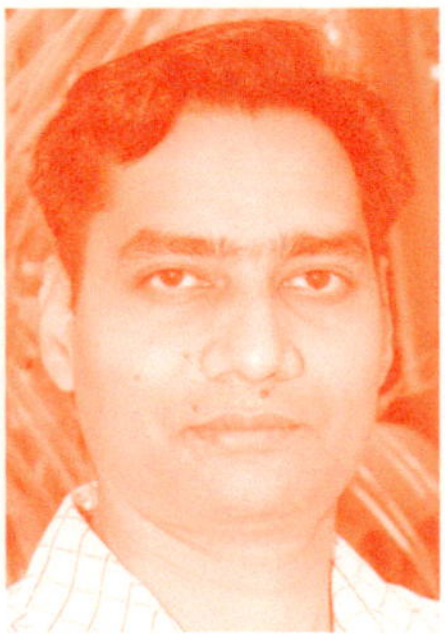
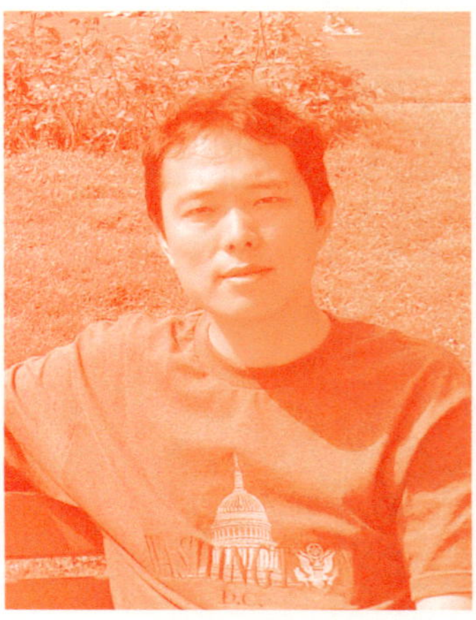
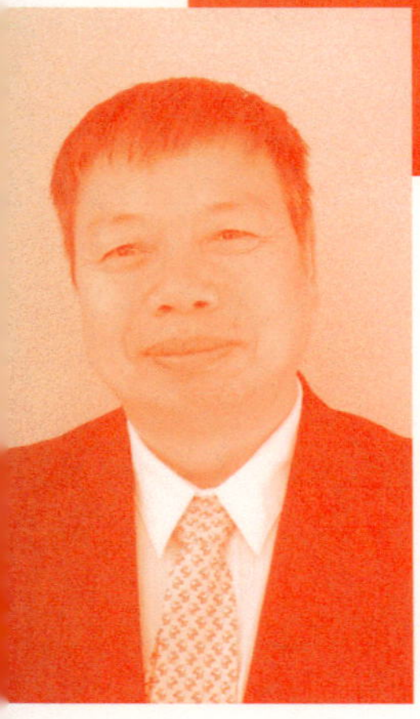
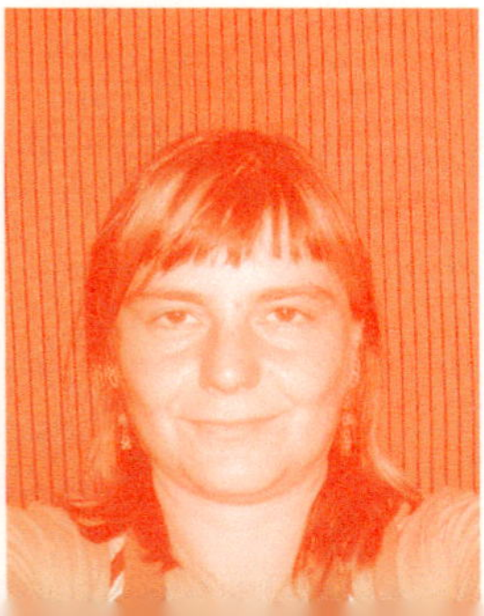

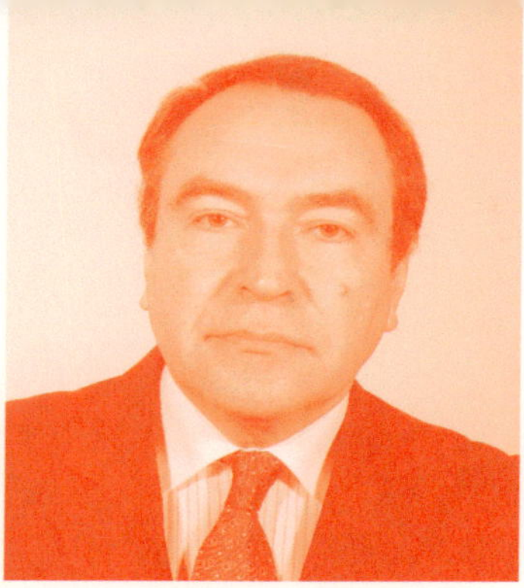
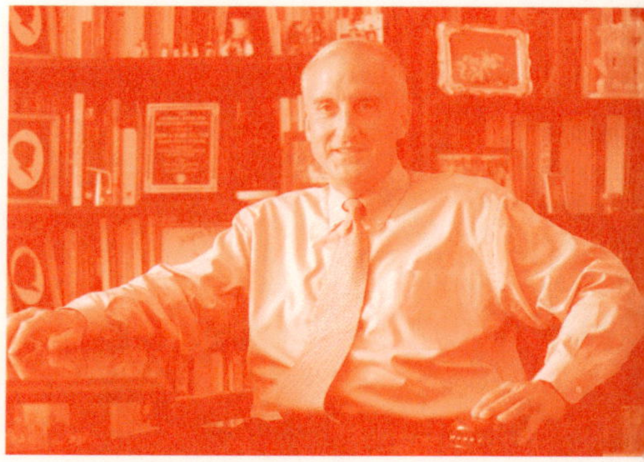
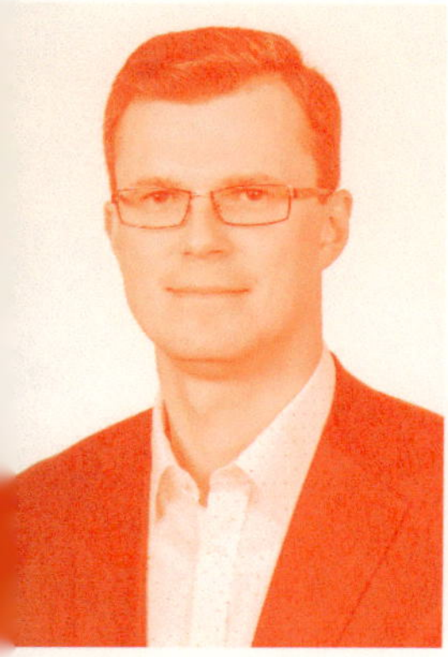
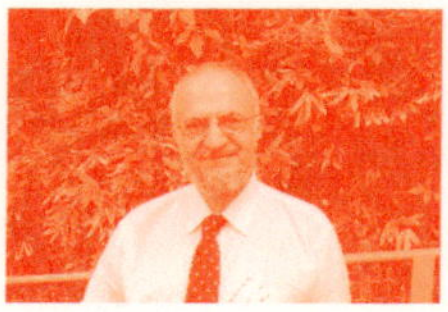
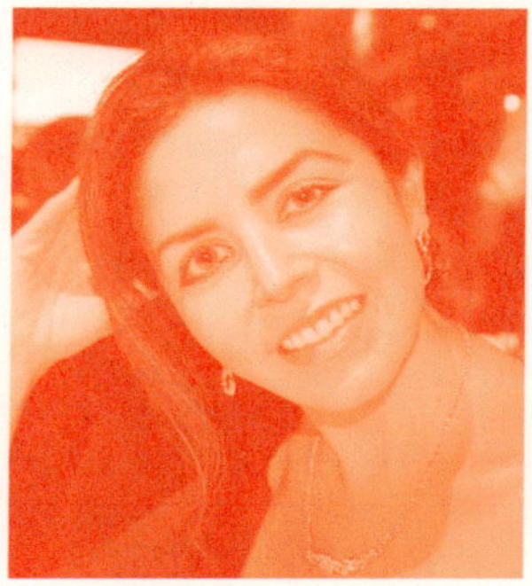

Supporting open minds since 2005

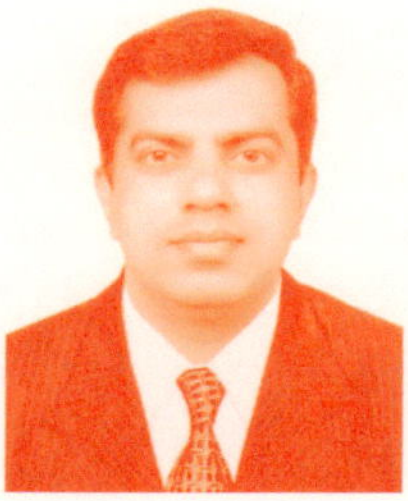
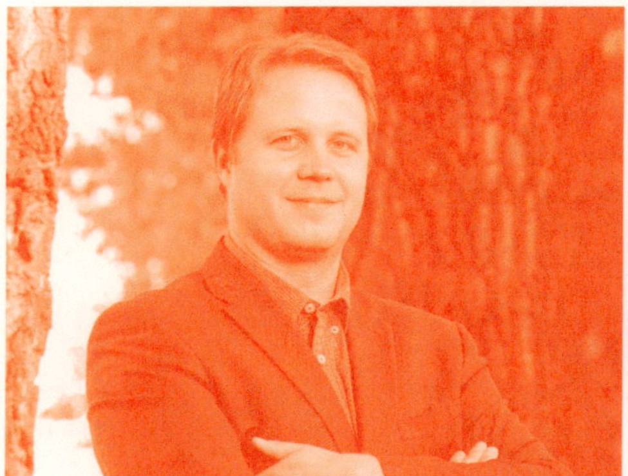
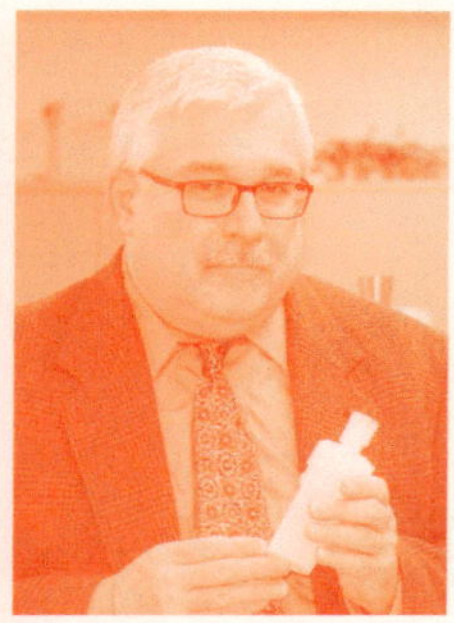
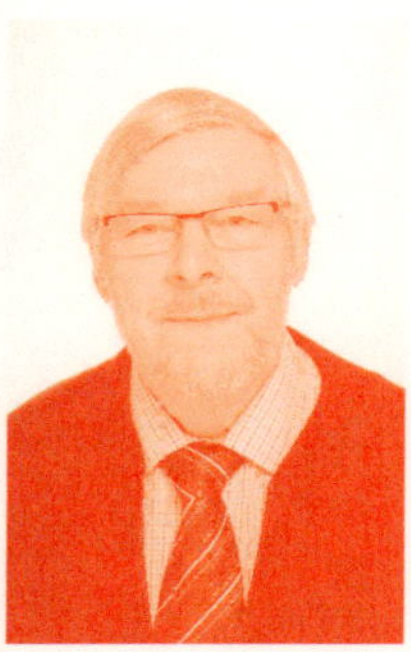
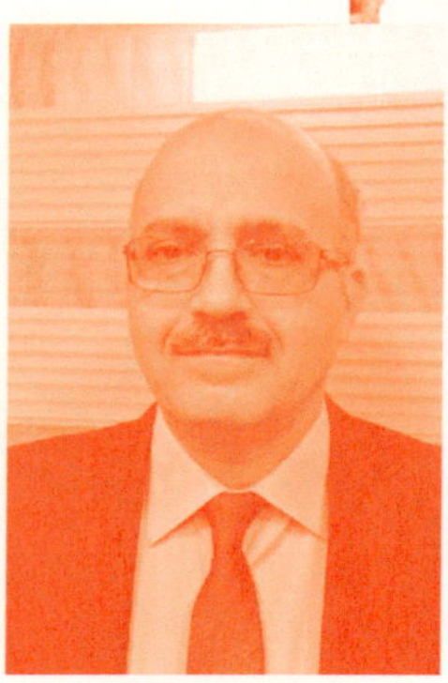
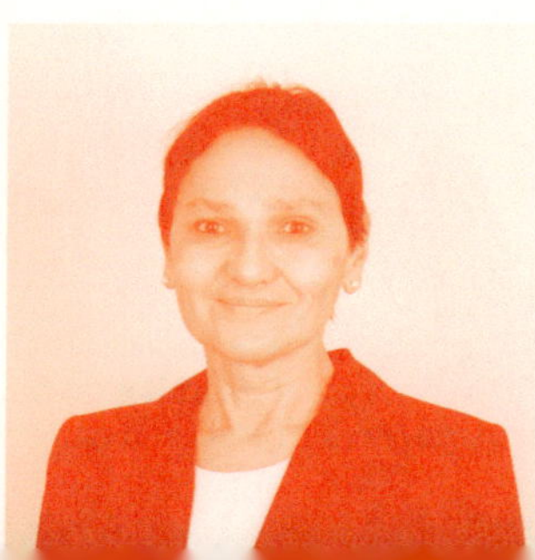
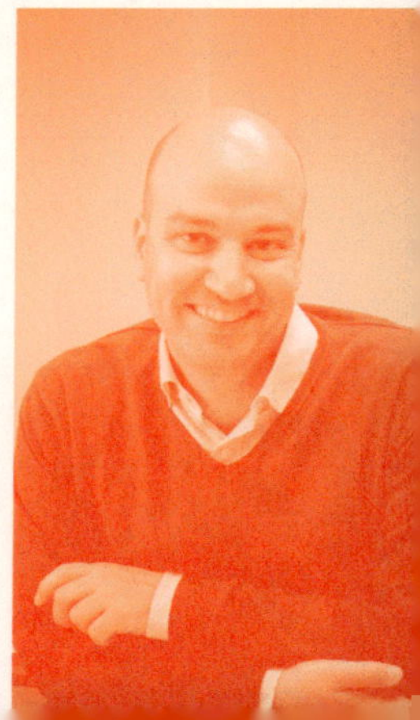

Skin Grafts for Successful Wound Closure
http://dx.doi.org/10.5772/intechopen.95174
Edited by Madhuri Gore

Contributors
Marcelo Fonseca, Aldo Cañete, Dino Ibaceta, Catalina Buchroithner, Florencia Disi, Juan Olivares, Rahul Gorka, Sundaram Ravanasamudram Rajaram, Gauthami Sundar, Ahmad Farouk Musa, Cheang Jia Min, Verónica Olvera-Cortés, Madhuri Gore

First published in London, United Kingdom, 2022 by IntechOpen
IntechOpen is the global imprint of INTECHOPEN LIMITED, registered in England and Wales, registration number: 11086078, 5 Princes Gate Court, London, SW7 2QJ, United Kingdom
Printed in Croatia

British Library Cataloguing-in-Publication Data
A catalogue record for this book is available from the British Library

Additional hard and PDF copies can be obtained from orders@intechopen.com

Skin Grafts for Successful Wound Closure
Edited by Madhuri Gore
p. cm.
Print ISBN 978-1-83969-746-3
Online ISBN 978-1-83969-747-0
eBook (PDF) ISBN 978-1-83969-748-7

For EU product safety concerns:
IN TECH d.o.o., Prolaz Marije Krucifikse Kozulić 3, 51000 Rijeka, Croatia, info@intechopen.com or visit our website at intechopen.com.

Meet the editor

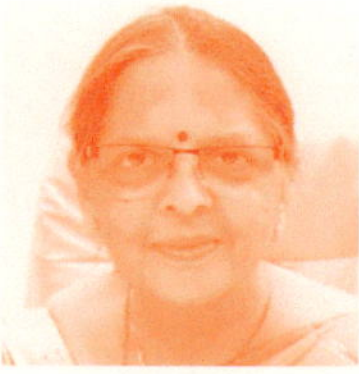

Dr. Madhuri Gore, a former Professor and Chief of Surgery at Lokmanya Tilak Municipal Medical College and General Hospital (LTMGH), India, is presently a consultant general surgeon in Mumbai, India. Her areas of interest are burns, non-burn trauma and wounds, and venous diseases. An acknowledged teacher and sought-after speaker, Dr. Gore established the first cadaver skin bank in India. She is an avid researcher and has been the chief investigator for more than twenty-five national and international clinical trials. She has more than seventy-five publications in national and international journals to her credit and has contributed seventeen chapters to various books. She has been honored with several awards, prizes, scholarships, and orations for her contribution to the fields of her special interest.

Contents

Preface

Wounds are common injuries that almost every human being experiences. They can vary in depth of tissue damage, etiology, location, contamination, lymphovascular integrity, and sensory neural function. They can be associated with diabetes, cardiovascular morbidity, hepatic and/or renal dysfunction, immunological status, malignancy, nutritional deficiencies, and so on. Wound healing is dependent on all these factors and many more.

Wounds that are limited to the epidermis and superficial layers of the dermis generally close and heal naturally. We now know the stages in this process and understand the role of multiple mediators, growth factors, cellular contributions, and the interaction between these components. However, there is no method by which we can control or modify this natural process of wound healing.

The situation is different when the wound involves full-thickness skin loss with or without loss of subcutaneous and deeper tissue. These wounds cannot achieve closure naturally, as both epidermal and dermal elements are lost. Without intervention, these wounds may remain as chronic, non-healing ulcers or they may close via wound contraction and formation of scar tissue causing functional limitations, deformities, and disfigurement. These scars may be unstable, leading to repeated breakdown, and are likely to develop Marjolin's ulcer, which is most often a squamous cell carcinoma of aggressive nature. Hence, a general recommendation is that wounds that do not close or that are not likely to close within 3–4 weeks of occurrence should be closed surgically with skin grafting or fasciocutaneous or myocutaneous flaps.

This book, *Skin Grafts for Successful Wound Closure*, focuses on various aspects related to free skin grafts; it does not address flaps. Skin autografts are necessary for providing permanent wound closure. While harvesting a split-thickness skin autograft from the appropriate donor area on the body of the patient, the surgeon is creating a partial-thickness wound that needs care for healing. Justifying this new wound and the pain and scarring associated with its healing requires a successful skin graft. Optimal preparation of the recipient wound bed is essential for the success of the graft take.

Section I, "Wound Bed Preparation," includes three chapters that elaborate on the different methods of wound bed preparation. The simultaneous management of systemic factors is necessary but is not within the purview of this publication.

The knowledge and practice of wound care are mandatory for all surgeons and thus every surgical trainee should know the basics as well as keep up with advances in the field of wound bed preparation and skin grafting procedures. As such, Chapter 1, "Preparation for a Successful Skin Grafting," in Section I describes various established methods for wound bed preparation. Although relatively new, negative pressure wound therapy is already well accepted and its efficacy has been illustrated in photographs. However, there is always a search for newer, better, easily available, and affordable topical agents, dressing materials, and techniques. Everything new requires evaluation and established methods need to be revalidated. Chapter 2, "Experience of Wound Bed Preparation with Different Methods," describes the experience of the author in evaluating a new topical agent and foam dressing prepared using new technology. It also describes the experience of using skin allografts and xenografts in a setting where the availability of both is uncommon. The chapter aims at providing stimulus for data collection, analysis, evaluation, and sharing of experiences about different methods of wound management. Chapter 3, "*Haruan* Extract (*Channa striatus*) as an Effective Mediator in Promoting Wound Healing," discusses a potential new method of wound healing using extract from Haruan, a carnivorous fish observed to have properties that are conducive to wound healing and pain relief. Research into the use of this extract is still in its infancy. The clinical trials described have not been designed to evaluate the effect of Haruan extract on wound healing or wound bed preparation. However, the extract's components and their actions suggest that this product has unevaluated promise in the field of wound bed preparation.

Once the recipient area is optimized to receive the skin autograft, the actual procedure needs to be performed with precision and planning. The planning process includes choice of the donor area, type of graft and its thickness, and processing and laying of the graft. Section II, "Skin Grafting," reviews the procedural aspects of skin grafting that are essential for the success of skin grafting procedures. Chapter 4, "Types of Skin Grafts," elaborates on the different types of skin grafts, provides guidance for choosing the correct graft, and discusses the procedure for skin graft harvesting and how to care for the donor site. It also gives information about methods of graft expansion and management of complications. This information is very valuable, particularly for surgeons undergoing training. Chapter 5, "Skin Graft Fixation and Methods," describes different methods of fixation of the skin graft over the wound bed. It is essential to maintain contact between these two surfaces, as hematoma, seroma, or movement of the graft over the wound bed can disturb nutrition to the graft in the initial period after the procedure. In the later phase of graft take, this can lead to poor uptake of the graft due to suboptimal vascularization of the applied skin graft thus compromising its survival. Chapter 6, "Procurement and Use of Cryopreserved Total Skin Allograft in Complex Wounds," describes a new concept of using a cryopreserved full-thickness skin allograft as an interim method in the process of achieving closure of complex wounds. In wounds with deep tissue loss over weight-bearing areas, a split-thickness skin graft may be inadequate in providing stable and robust wound closure due to a lack of adequate thickness of the dermis. Use of an acellular dermis or dermal regeneration template are other alternatives available in such a situation. Use of full-thickness allograft skin obtained from redundant skin excised during abdominoplasty and cryopreserved after complete defatting appears to be an effective alternative for providing neodermis over complex wounds. If more workers in the field of wound care start using this technique, it will allow for establishing the utility of this method in a more convincing way.

The opportunity to edit this book has given me the pleasure of acquainting myself with the contributions of other experts in the field of wound care. I enjoyed the experience thoroughly. I hope readers will find this book a useful resource and that its contents spur further interest and research in the field.

I wish to express my very special thanks to Author Service Manager Ms. Mia Vulovic at IntechOpen for all the support she provided throughout the editorial process. My very sincere thanks to the complete publishing team.

Dr. Madhuri Gore
Consultant Surgeon,
Zen Hospital,
Chembur, Mumbai, India

Section 1

Wound Bed Preparation

Chapter 1

Preparation for a Successful Skin Grafting

Rahul Gorka

Abstract

In this chapter, we shall look into the pre-requisites for a successful skin grafting. This includes patient selection, identifying various factors—patient related, environment related, treatment related, and optimizing them for a successful outcome. Avoiding/removing the adverse factors and improving the wound bed environment require knowledge, experience, and checklist to be followed, so as not to miss any of these pre-requisites. This would ensure complete take of the skin graft, with good reconstructive and esthetic outcome. Various factors include patients' general health, comorbidities, etiology of wound, duration and contamination, granulation tissue, local wound blood supply, wound sepsis, edema, vascular disease, wound bacteriology culture sensitivity, etc. The ultimate goal of improving success of skin grafting will lead to early recovery of patient, reducing hospital stay, burden on health infrastructure, and reduced loss of workdays, thereby reducing the socioeconomic impact of wound.

Keywords: skin grafting, optimizing, wound bed, graft-take, outcome

1. Introduction

Several factors have to be considered before planning a skin grafting. This ensures achievement of optimal tissue environment at the wound site. The quality of wound bed has to be enhanced so as to ensure a successful "take" of the skin graft. The donor site area skin color, thickness, and mechanical property should preferably match the recipient site skin quality. The causes of poor skin graft include multiple factors such as chronic or insufficiently debrided wounds, poorly vascularized wound bed, or high bacterial load.

2. Recipient site considerations

2.1 Wound bed preparation

Wound bed preparation is a valuable concept that attempts to systematize the approach to the treatment of chronic wounds [1]. The "take" of skin graft depends on a healthy well-vascularized wound bed. It is supported by an adequate quantity of blood vessels near the surface. Appropriate skin graft take is not allowed in ischemic, previously irradiated and scar tissues, bone, and tendon, as they have an insufficient blood supply.

Consistency of necrotic tissue also varies as tissue damage worsens/deepens:

- Slough: yellow/tan, thin, mucinous, or stringy (partial thickness damage)
- Eschar: brown/black, soft of hard (full-thickness damage)

We should assess the wound using a validated wound assessment tool such as the Bates-Jensen Wound Assessment tool [2]. Skin grafting can be done in the presence of well-vascularized peritendon and periosteum. Marginal wound re-epithelization is seen to occur in chronic wounds, which grows into the tissue and interrupts the lateral reconnections of the graft. Hence, it is advisable to do sharp excision of the margins with a blade before grafting.

Quantitatively, the bacterial level must be less than 10^5 bacteria per gram of tissue for a successful skin grafting. Clinically, the wound should be "clean" and debrided of all necrotic tissues. The chief aims of treatment should be the control of the infection and the promotion of the natural processes of healing [3]. The necrotic tissue debris physically impedes and chemically decelerates ingrowth of blood vessels into the skin graft. Necrotic tissue and slough are the key contributors to wound chronicity, and thus, debridement is necessary for wound healing [4]. Those wounds that are left open for many days contain heavy bacterial contamination and therefore need to be substantially debrided before skin grafting. Sharp debridement leads to the release of cytokines and mediators of inflammation [5]. The various debridement techniques [6] used to prepare the recipient site include the following:

Debridement Type	**Definition**	**Examples**
Mechanical	Use of external mechanical method for debridement of necrotic tissue	Wet-to-dry gauze, water spray, whirlpool, wound wash
Enzymatic	Use of topical agent containing proteolytic enzyme which can help slough separation	Collagenase Papain urea
Surgical	Surgical debridement of necrotic tissue using sharp instruments	Scalpel, scissor, curette
Autolytic	Separation of necrotic tissue by natural process due to proteolytic enzymes liberated by wound surface and bacteria colonizing the wound	hydrocolloids,, hydrogels, alginates, hypertonic dressings aid autolytic process
Biologic	Use of medical grade maggots to achieve wound debridement	Larval debridement therapy [7]

Conservative Sharp Wound Debridement (CSWD) is a suitable method of debridement when there is dead necrotic tissue such as slough or eschar, callus-tissue around the wound, or hyperkeratosis (which is clearly demarcated from the healthy tissue, where other types of debridement may not give optimum result and/or where speed is essential) [2].

It has been understood that a "granulating" wound has better chances of skin graft take. Active bleeding of the wound bed can lead to hematoma collection under the graft, thereby inhibiting graft take. Adequate hemostasis can be performed using electrocautery and suture ligation.

Before skin grafting, the surrounding soft tissue can be adjusted to cover critical structures such as tendons or bones if they are exposed without peritendon or periosteum. A moist wound environment has been shown to accelerate wound healing by up to 50% compared with exposure to air [8]. Vacuum-assisted closure therapy or dermal substitutes can be used to prepare small areas of tendons and bones, by growing granulation tissue from the sides.

2.2 Functional consideration

An optimum skin graft can give a good functional and esthetic skin reconstruction. Particular attention should be given to the size of graft needed, the degree of wound contraction anticipated, the color and texture of the skin required, and the need for adnexal glands. More the amount of dermis in the skin graft, lesser is the amount of wound contraction.

Full-thickness grafts provide excellent cosmetic results since they include the complete epidermis and dermis and thereby have minimal contraction. Full-thickness skin grafts are commonly used for syndactyly release, nipple-areola reconstruction, or ectropion release. Full-thickness graft donor site is limited and can be increased by tissue expansion before harvesting.

The donor sites of very thin skin grafts like epidermal grafts heal quickly with minimal contraction, but do not resist the recipient wound contraction. This is desirable on areas such as large scalp wounds and abdominal wounds, where wound contraction leads to gradual pulling of the wound edges together, reducing the skin graft requirement. In a second stage surgery, the contracted skin graft can be excised and the wound can be primarily closed to get better functional and esthetic results. The skin thickness varies from upper eyelid (thin) to trunk and leg (thick).

2.3 Esthetic considerations

The final appearance of skin graft color is dependent upon skin texture, melanin pigmentation, and blood flow. According to Gillies' principles, like should replace like. So the replacement of tissue from a similar or surrounding site gives the best color match [9]. For face, full-thickness skin grafts are preferred from sites such as supraclavicular, posterior auricular, upper eyelid, or scalp [10]. For nipple-areola complex, skin grafts from the contralateral areola or genitalia may be used. Glabrous skin grafts from hypothenar area can be placed over palms and soles of feet.

3. Conclusion

Preparation for a successful skin grafting entails the optimization of patient factors including systemic and local tissue environment, in addition to

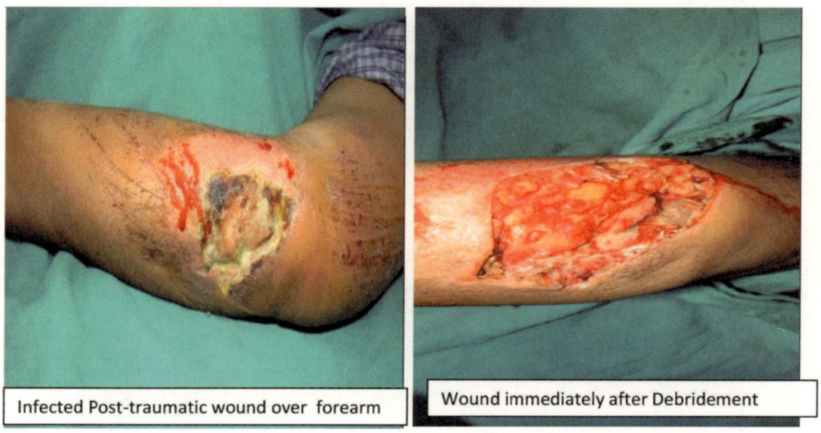

Figure 1.
Foreaarm Infected wound management by debridement followed by NPWT dressings and Skin grafting.

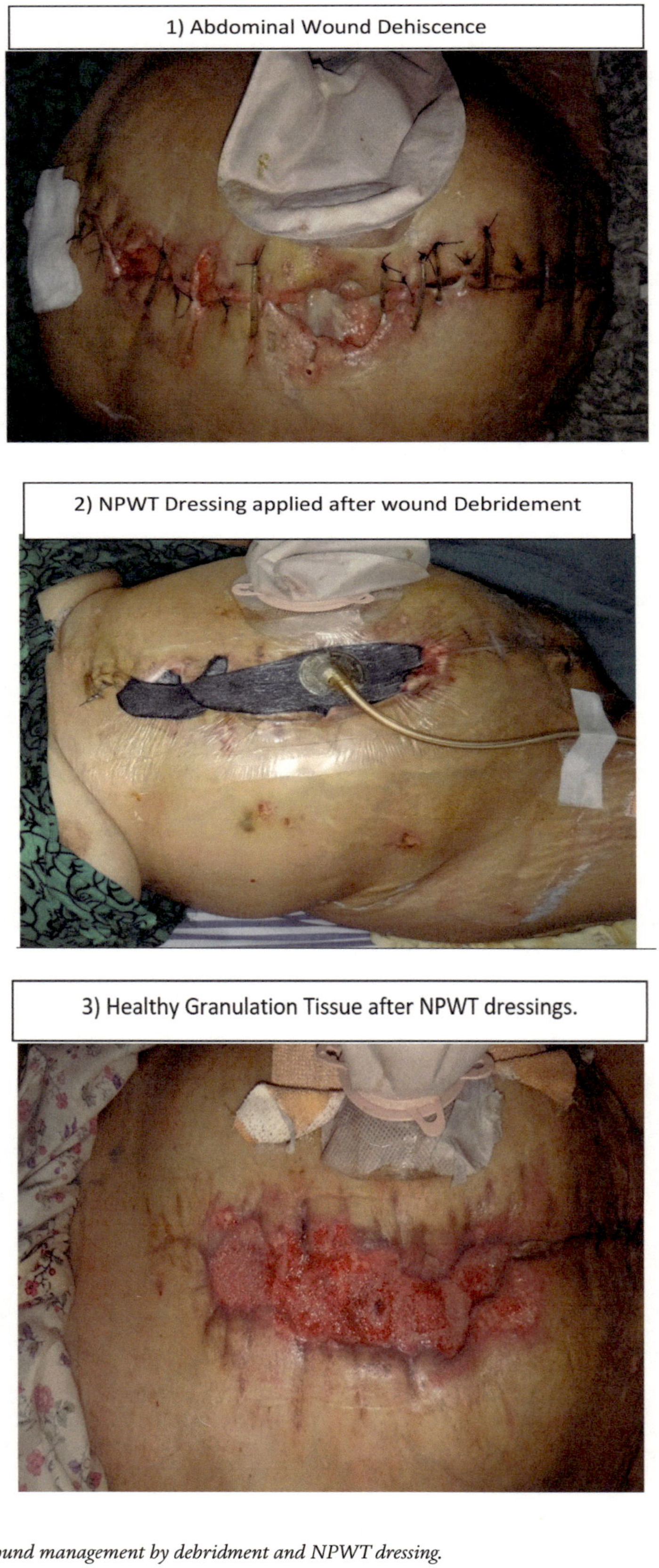

Figure 2.
Abdominal wound management by debridment and NPWT dressing.

DOI: http://dx.doi.org/10.5772/intechopen.101375

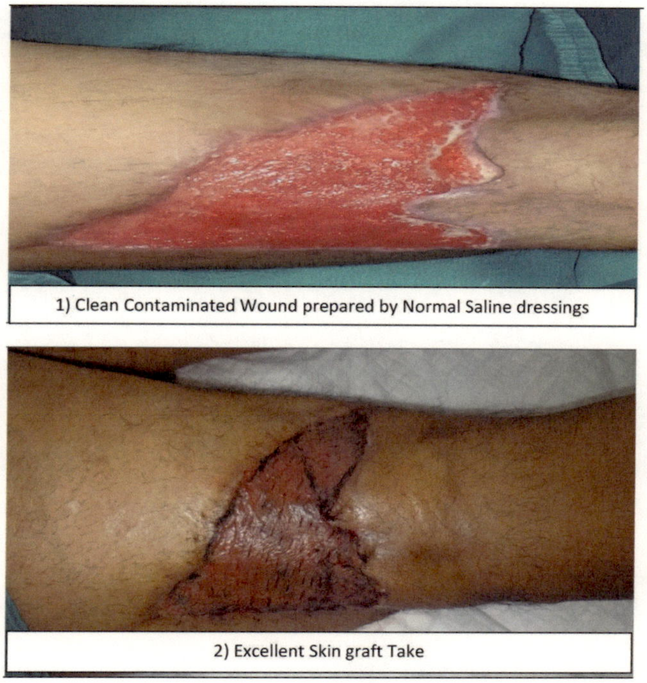

Figure 3.
Thigh wound bed preparation by noormal saline dressings.

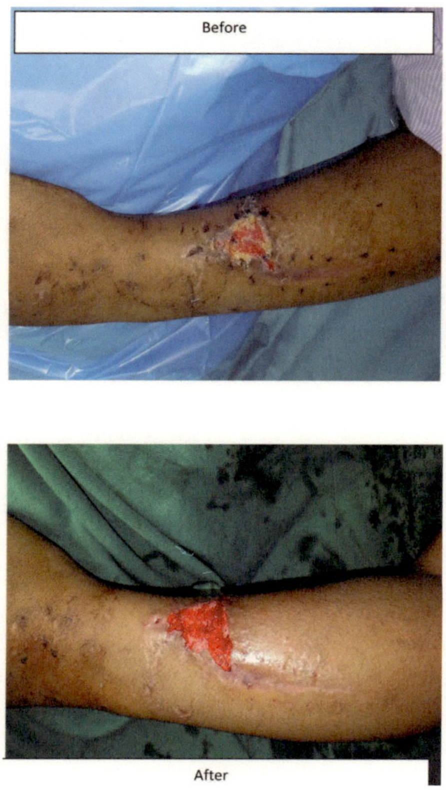

Figure 4.
Forearm wound preparation by topical antibiotic ointments.

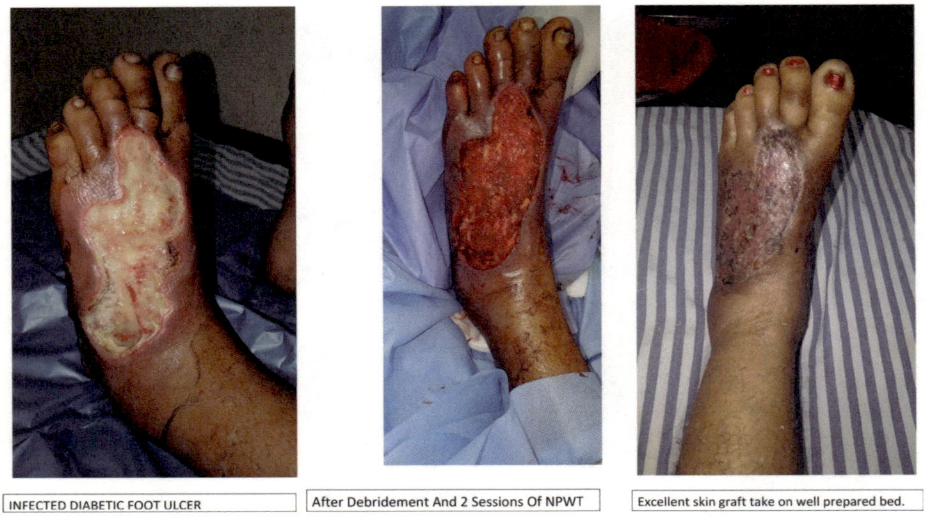

Figure 5.
Diabetic foot wound bed preparation.

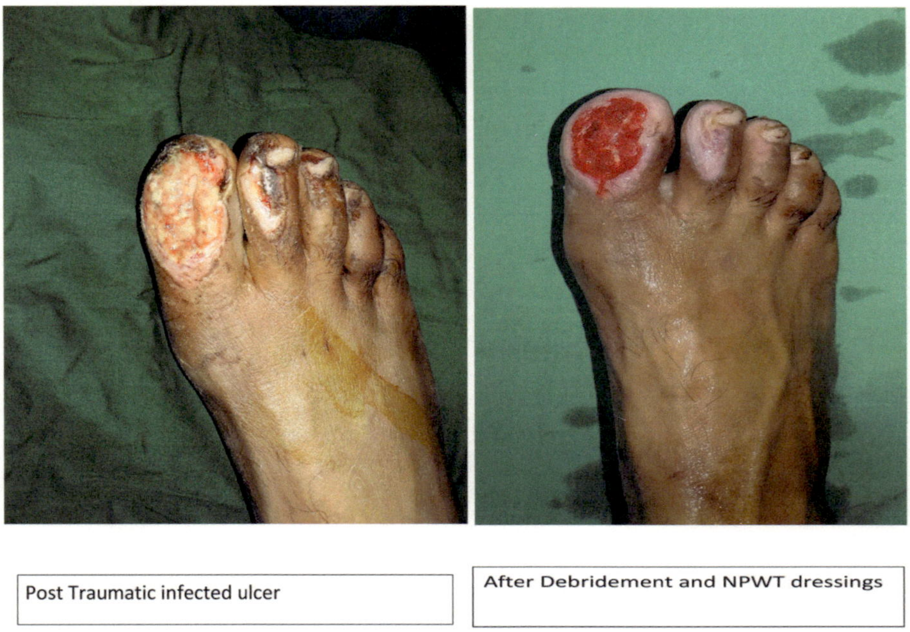

Figure 6.
Great toe raw area wound preparation by debridement and NPWT.

consideration of functional and esthetic factors. The author has experienced that the simpler techniques of mechanical as well as sharp surgical debridement followed by negative pressure wound therapy in appropriately selected patients (as shown in **Figures 1–8**) fetch almost cent percent skin graft take results, with both functional and esthetic targets achieved.

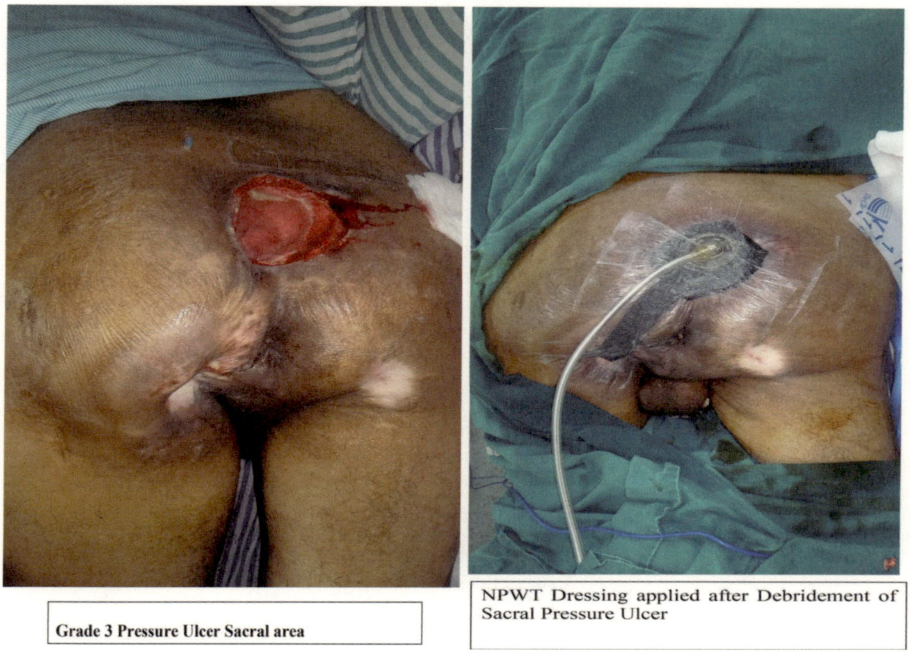

Figure 7.
NPWT dressing for pressure ulcers.

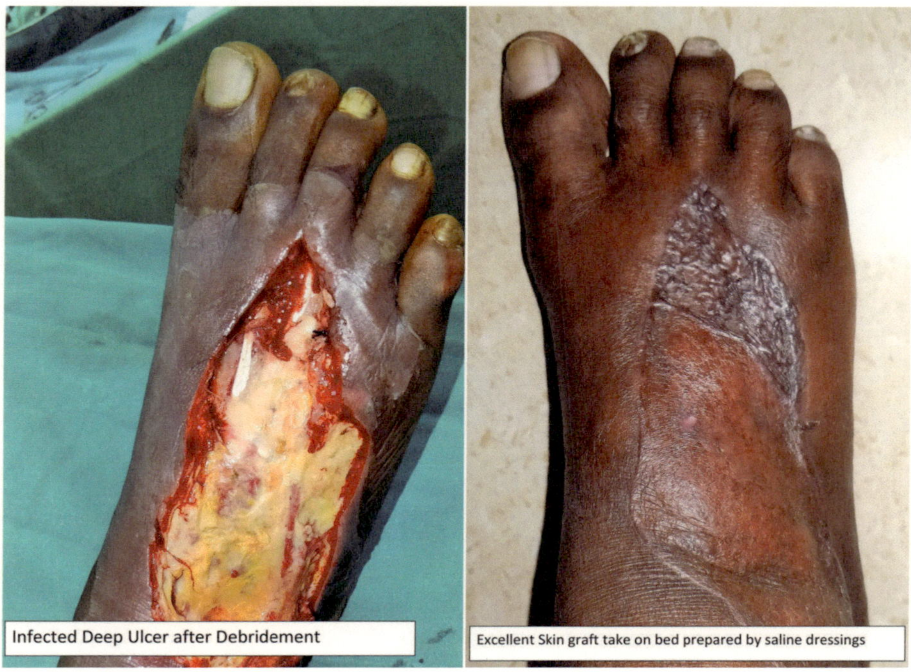

Figure 8.
Diabetic foot ulcer- wound bed preparation by debridement and normal saline dressings.

Conflict of interest

The authors declare no conflict of interest.

Author details

Rahul Gorka
Department of Burns, Plastic and Reconstructive Surgery, Government Medical College Jammu, India

*Address all correspondence to: rahulgorka8@gmail.com

References

[1] Schultz G, Sibbald R, Falanga V, Ayello E, Dowsett C, Harding K, et al. Wound bed preparation: A systematic approach to wound management. Wound Repair and Regeneration: Official Publication of the Wound Healing Society [and] the European Tissue Repair Society. 2003;**11**(Suppl. 1): S1-S28

[2] Harris C, Coutts P, Raizman R, Grady N. Sharp wound debridement: Patient selection and perspectives. CWCMR. 2018;**6**:29-36

[3] Guo S, Dipietro LA. Factors affecting wound healing. Journal of Dental Research. 2010;**89**(3):219-229. DOI: 10.1177/0022034509359125

[4] Percival SL, Suleman L. Slough and biofilm: Removal of barriers to wound healing by desloughing. Journal of Wound Care. 2015;**24**(11):498-510

[5] Milne J. Wound-bed preparation: The importance of rapid and effective desloughing to promote healing. The British Journal of Nursing. 2015; **24**(Sup. 20):S52-S58

[6] Sibbald RG, Williamson D, Orsted HL, Campbell K, Keast D, Krasner D, et al. Preparing the wound bed--debridement, bacterial balance, and moisture balance. Ostomy/Wound Management. 2000;**46**(11):14-22. 24-8, 30-5; quiz 36-7

[7] Growth Effects of Phaenicia Sericata Larval Extracts on Fibroblasts: Mechanism for Wound Healing by Maggot Therapy - ScienceDirect [Internet]. [Cited 2021 October 15]. Available from: https://www.sciencedirect.com/science/article/abs/pii/S0024320596006881?via%3Dihub

[8] Geronemus RG, Robins P. The effect of two new dressings on epidermal wound healing. The Journal of Dermatologic Surgery and Oncology. 1982;**8**(10):850-852

[9] Shimizu R, Kishi K. Skin Graft. Plastic Surgery International. 2012; **2012**:1-5

[10] Thornton JF. Skin grafts and skin substitutes. Selected Readings in Plastic Surgery. 2004;**10**(1):78

Chapter 2

Experience of Wound Bed Preparation with Different Methods

Madhuri Gore

Abstract

The ultimate goal of wound care is to obtain wound closure either by natural process or by use of surgical technique and so all the steps need to be taken with a plan to reach the goal at the earliest. While performing skin grafting, closure of the existing wound is the aim, but the procedure also creates another wound (though superficial), causes pain, and may have healing issues. Optimal bed preparation is mandatory to obtain successful uptake of skin graft and to avoid loss of precious skin autograft. Every wound has its own unique needs and demands. Different agents and methods are often needed to meet these demands. It is essential to accrue experience and develop insight into the efficacy, utility, and advantages of different approaches for wound bed preparation. The availability, cost of the method, socioeconomic status of the patient, type of health care system, ease of access to facility, expertise—all these and many other factors play a role in deciding the choice of method for wound bed preparation. It is possible that different methods may be developed, evaluated, and found to be useful in different countries or different parts of the same country too. The author has evaluated methods spread over a wide spectrum including indigenously prepared topical agent, barrier foam dressing prepared using advanced technology, porcine xenografts which are not available in India, and skin allografts from the very first skin bank in India set up by the author and colleagues. The experience shared here looks at the ability of the method to control infection, inflammation, pain besides the time taken to achieve effective wound bed preparation and frequency of dressing change needed, along with ease of training.

Keywords: wound bed, topical agent, porcine xenografts, skin allografts, barrier foam dressing, control of infection, inflammation, skin autograft success, wound closure

1. Introduction

The aim of treating a patient with a wound is to correct the systemic factors and to achieve wound closure, either by natural processes or by using surgical techniques. To achieve this end concept of wound bed preparation was proposed by Dr. Falanga and Dr. Sibbald in the year 2000 [1] and updated thereafter. Besides controlling systemic aberrations such as cardiac failure, diabetes mellitus, liver or renal dysfunction, vascular insufficiency, etc., successful management of the wound environment needs thorough understanding and assessment of multiple factors related to the wound. The components that need attention include the following [1].

1. Tissue management

2. Infection and inflammation management

3. Moisture balance

4. Epithelial advancement

The author has had a long association with wounds—burn and nonburn. Besides developing a simple, cheap, and easily available dressing for wounds [2], the author had the opportunity to conduct clinical trials to evaluate new topical agents, wound dressings and xenografts and skin allografts and their role in wound bed preparation. Some of these studies have been published and some are being shared here for the first time. It is hoped that this may provide a stimulus for research in the field of wound bed preparation.

A full-thickness wound that is not likely to achieve closure by natural process or secondary suturing, or is likely to cause esthetic/functional issues if left to heal on its own by secondary intention, needs skin grafting to achieve wound closure. Hence while assessing the efficacy of a new tool in achieving optimal wound bed preparation, it is essential to evaluate the following factors -

1. Time taken to achieve wound status ready to receive skin graft -This includes separation of necrotic tissue, infection control, relief from inflammation and edema, satisfactory vascularization, and healthy granulation.

2. Success of skin grafting procedure.

3. Availability and cost of the agent/method under evaluation.

Observations such as relief of pain, ease, and conformability of dressing, frequency of dressing change, absence of toxicity, allergy; ease of training family members about the performance of wound care procedures are other important considerations.

Though it would be ideal to have a controlled trial, the presence of multiple variables affecting wound response, makes it very difficult to have absolutely comparable study and control groups. The study related to the topical agent being shared here, in brief, is unpublished data.

2. Topical agent: Panchvalkal

2.1 The product

It is hot ethanolic extract of barks of five trees added to liquefied petroleum jelly. The names of the trees are Ficus Bengalensis, Ficus Religiosa, Ficus Infectoria, Ficus Glomerata, and Azadirachta Indica.

It was shown to have broad-spectrum antimicrobial activity which included *Staphylococcus aureus*, *Pseudomonas Aeruginosa*, *Escherichia coli*, Proteus V, Streptococcous Pyo., anaerobes.

Studies related to mutagenicity, skin toxicity, oral toxicity, mucus membrane irritation revealed the product to be safe.

2.2 The study

To evaluate the efficacy and safety of Panchvalkal as topical agent for wound dressing.

After obtaining approval from the institutional ethics committee, an open-labeled clinical trial was conducted in 2003 enrolling 100 patients with wounds after obtaining informed consent.

Initial surgical debridement was performed when needed. The wound was cleaned with normal saline. The topical agent under evaluation was applied over the wound and covered with paraffin impregnated tulle gras. This was covered with secondary dressing of gamjee and fixed with appropriate method (bandage or tape). The dressing was changed every alternate day and the wound was evaluated for slough, exudate, pain, inflammation along with wound photograph at regular intervals. The time taken to reach endpoint was noted. The endpoint was readiness for skin grafting, secondary suturing, wound closure by contraction, and/or epithelization.

The results have been provided here in brief (unpublished data). There were 73 males and 27 females included in the study. The mean age of the patients was 39.71 years with range of 13 to 75 years. The most frequent cause of the wound was complex skin and soft tissue infection (CSSTI) (**Table 1**) including abscess, necrotizing fascitis. Surgical site infection or guillotine amputation stump, fresh burns were the causes of wounds in 23 patients.

In 43 out of 100 enrolled patients, the wounds were sterile at the time of entry in the trial and this included patients with fresh burns, postoperative wound gapes, and some bed sores. These wounds continued to remain sterile at the end of the study. In 57 patients wounds grew various pathogens at the time of entry in the study. *S. aureus* and *P. aeruginosa* were the most common isolates, followed by Klebsiella, Proteus, *E. coli*, and then Acinetobacter in a few. In 24 of 57 patients (42.1%) the wound became sterile before the endpoint was reached. The remaining wounds swab cultures grew *P. aeruginosa* and Klebsiella. None of the wounds grew Streptococci at any time in the study. Reduction of edema, wound discharge, slough, pain are all indicators of control of infection and related inflammation.

Etiology	No. of patients
CSSTI	47
SSI	23
Injury—Nonburn	17
Burn injury	13
Total	100

Table 1.
Wound Etiology (topical agent).

Time in days	Depth of wound	No. of patients
Within 7 days	Full-thickness	45
Between 7 and 14 days	Full + mixed depth thickness	31
More than 14 days	Full + Partial thickness	24
Total		100

Table 2.
Time taken to reach endpoint (topical agent).

Wound depth	STSG	Epithelization	Contraction	Secondary suturing	Total
Full-thickness	67	Nil	14	11	92
Mixed depth	3	3	Nil	Nil	6
Superficial	0	2	Nil	Nil	2
Total	70	5	14	11	100

Table 3.
Method of wound closure (topical agent).

Tables 2 and **3** provide the observations about the time taken to reach endpoint and methods used to achieve wound closure. Total 70 wounds out of 100 required split-thickness skin grafting (STSG) to achieve wound closure and 45 of these had reached the endpoint in less than 7 days and the remaining 31 were ready for STSG by 14 days. The graft take was complete in 66 of 70 (94.3%) wounds and in 4 cases partial graft loss was noted. This indicates good graft bed preparation.

2.3 Conclusions

1. Significant reduction in wound slough, exudate from the wound, abatement in the signs of inflammation such as edema (**Figure 1a–c**), pain was noted from as early as the second day of starting the application of topical agent under trial. The difference between these parameters at enrollment and at the endpoint was statistically significant with $p < 0.05$.

2. The agent was found to be suitable for diabetic foot wounds too (**Figure 2a** and **b**).

3. The successful take of skin graft (94.3%) indicates that the wound bed preparation achieved was optimal in terms of wound vascularization as well as infection control.

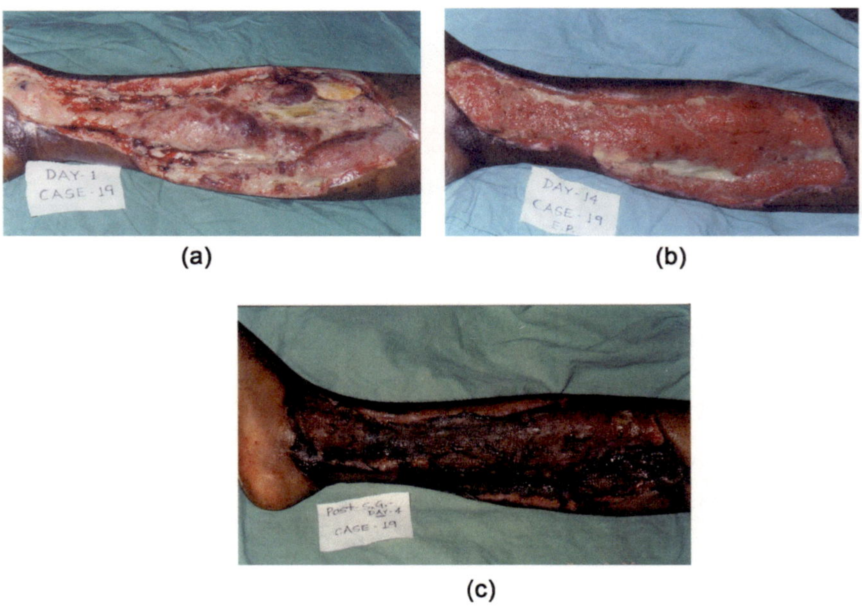

Figure 1.
a. Necrotising fasciitis after surgical debridement. b. Wound at endpoint on day 14. c: After skin grafting.

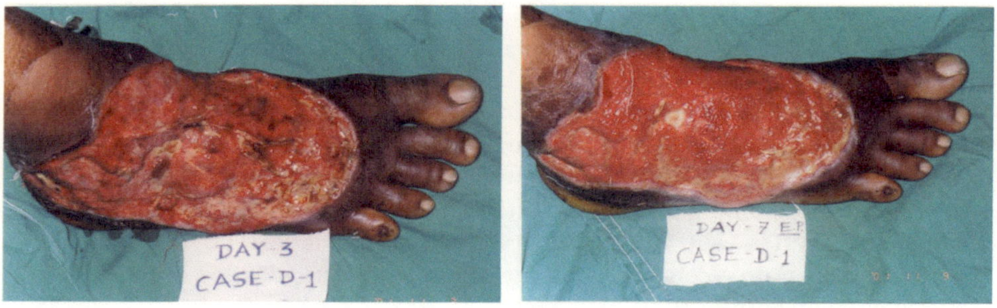

(a) (b)

Figure 2.
a. Diabetic foot ulcer. b. Ulcer at endpoint.

4. No side effects, local reactions were noted and the topical agent was well tolerated by the patients.

This study led to commercial preparation (Treval) of this topical agent and the use could be continued. But due to the inadequate availability of appropriate quality barks of necessary trees, the preparation of the product had to be stopped in a year or two. We lost an indigenously prepared natural product with good efficacy for wound bed preparation.

3. Porcine xenograft

Porcine xenograft has been used for wound bed preparation with the hope of improving the take of skin autograft over burn and nonburn wounds [3, 4]. A recently published article [5] compared the use of porcine xenografts with no specific method for wound bed preparation and concluded that there was no difference in these two methods in terms of wound closure. But the author's experience differs from this study.

Though porcine xenografts are in use for wound management in many countries, these are not available in India for regular use. There is no published report from India about the use of porcine xenografts over different types of wounds. Hence, it is important to share this Indian experience about use of porcine xenografts.

A randomized controlled trial was conducted at LTM Medical college and general hospital by the author and colleagues in 2009–2010 after approval from the institutional ethics committee. The unpublished data of this clinical trial is being shared here. After randomization of the patients, the type of wound care the patient was to receive was explained to the patient in detail and informed consent was obtained. None of the patients enrolled in the study group refused to accept the porcine xenograft.

3.1 Clinical trial—Comparison between Porcine Xenograft and usual wound dressing for wound bed preparation—A randomized controlled trial

3.1.1 Study design and protocol

Patients with wounds on any part of the body were randomized to study (Porcine xenograft (PX)) or to control (usual dressing (UD)) group. The presence of diabetes mellitus was not an exclusion criterion.

Porcine xenograft is not commercially available in India. So, full-thickness porcine skin was procured from the abattoir after the pig was stunned and then skinned as is the usual procedure there. This skin was brought to the laboratory in the department and split-thickness skin grafts were taken with all aseptic precautions using Humby's handle and blade. The grafts were treated with antibiotics (Crystalline penicillin + Gentamycin) and then preserved in 85% Glycerol following the same method as used for skin allograft preservation. These porcine xenografts were used as required by washing them with normal saline till soft. Grafts were covered with paraffin impregnated gauze after application on the wound. Secondary dressing and fixation were with Gamgee and bandage or tape.

The control group received wound dressing with the application of topical agents such as povidone Iodine ointment or Framycetin cream covered by primary nonadherent (impregnated tulle gras) and secondary dressing and bandage or tape fixation.

3.2 Results

The wound parameters evaluated were same as described in the previous experience with Panchvalkal topical agent. The epidemiological data has been provided in **Table 4**. It reveals that the study and control groups were comparable in all aspects such as age and gender of patients, location of body parts involved, etiology of wounds, presence of exudate. The commonest comorbidity observed in both groups was diabetes mellitus. Other comorbid conditions observed in both groups were hypertension, ischemic heart disease, tuberculosis, addiction to smoking and these were comparable between the two groups. The difference in the duration of symptoms was not statistically significant.

The observations at the endpoint (which was the readiness of the wound to receive STSG) have been presented in **Table 5**. The difference observed in the reduction in wound size at the endpoint was not statistically significant. The wounds in the study group treated with porcine xenografts achieved better microbial clearance as compared to the control group. At the endpoint, 15 out of 30 wounds in PX group and 6 out of 30 wounds in the UD group did not grow any organisms on culture (**Table 6**). This difference was statistically significant. At enrollment, the isolates grown from the wounds in PX group were *E. coli*, MRSA, Pseudomonas, and Klebsiella. At the endpoint, no wounds in PX group had a

Characters	Study group (PX) 30 patients	Control group (UD) 30 patients
Age range and mean	20 to 60 yrs. (41.7 yrs)	20 to 63 yrs. (40.7 yrs)
Men	22	25
Women	8	5
Extremity involvement	25	22
Other body parts	5	8
Burn & non-burn trauma	12	11
Infective & other wounds	18	19
Seropurulant exudate	22	23
No exudate	8	7
Diabetes mellitus	14	16
Duration of symptoms (Mean)	17.7 Days	8.3 Days

Table 4.
Epidemiological data of study and control group (PX and UD).

Results	Study group (PX) 30 pts Number of patients (%)	Control group (UD) 30 pts Number of patients (%)
Reduction in wound size	22 (73.3%)	20 (66.6%)
No microbial growth	15 (50%)	6 (20%)*
Clearance of slough	28 (93.4%)	25 (83.3%)
Reduction in pain score VAS	3.83 (Mean)	1.26 (Mean)*
Days to reach endpoint	8.66 days (Mean)	12.7 days (Mean)*

*VAS – Visual analog scale * P value <0.05 Significant.*

Table 5.
Presentation of observations at the endpoint (PX and UD).

Microbial Culture	Study group 30 pts (PX) Enrollment	Study group 30 pts(PX) Endpoint	Control group 30 pts (UD) Enrollment	Control group 30 pts (UD) Endpoint
No isolate	8 (26.6%)	15 (50%)	7 (23.3%)	6 (20%)*
Polymicrobial	2	0	5	3
Monomicrobial	20 (66.6%)	15 (50%)	18 (60%)	21 (70%)
Total	30	30	30	30

** P value <0.05 Significant.*

Table 6.
Outcome of microbial culture at entry and endpoint (PX and UD).

polymicrobial infection and the organism grown from 15 wounds were Proteus in 10 and Acinetobacter in 5. In UD group at enrollment 18 wounds and at endpoint 21 wounds showed growth of single isolates. These included Klebsiella, Pseudomonas, MSSA, *E. coli* at enrollment and Proteus, MRSA, Acinetobacter, and *E. coli* at the end point. No wound showed the presence of streptococci at endpoint. The initial pain score was comparable in both study (6.83) and control (6.66) group. But the reduction in pain score indicating relief of pain was statistically significant in the study (PX) group as compared to the control group. The mean number of days required to reach the endpoint were 8.66 in study group and 12.7 days in the control group (**Figure 3a** and **b**). This difference was statistically significant.

3.3 Conclusion

This study suggested that in comparison to the usual wound dressing the wound bed preparation was achieved earlier, with a significant reduction in pain and control of microbial load when porcine xenograft was applied over the wounds. An associated benefit was the reduction in the frequency of dressing change in the study group. The patients had to be admitted in the hospital or had to attend an outpatient clinic for a dressing change. Porcine xenografts were accepted by all patients randomized to study group.

In 86% of the patients in study group xenograft adherence to the wound bed was noted. But the xenograft uptake (vascularization) was not noted in any wound. Chiu and Burd [4] observed that adherence of porcine xenograft to the wound is related to its antimicrobial action. Adherence thus indicates the possibility of subsequent improvement in skin autograft take.

Raimer and colleagues [6] found porcine xenografts to be useful in the management of wounds following Mohs micrographic surgical procedures.

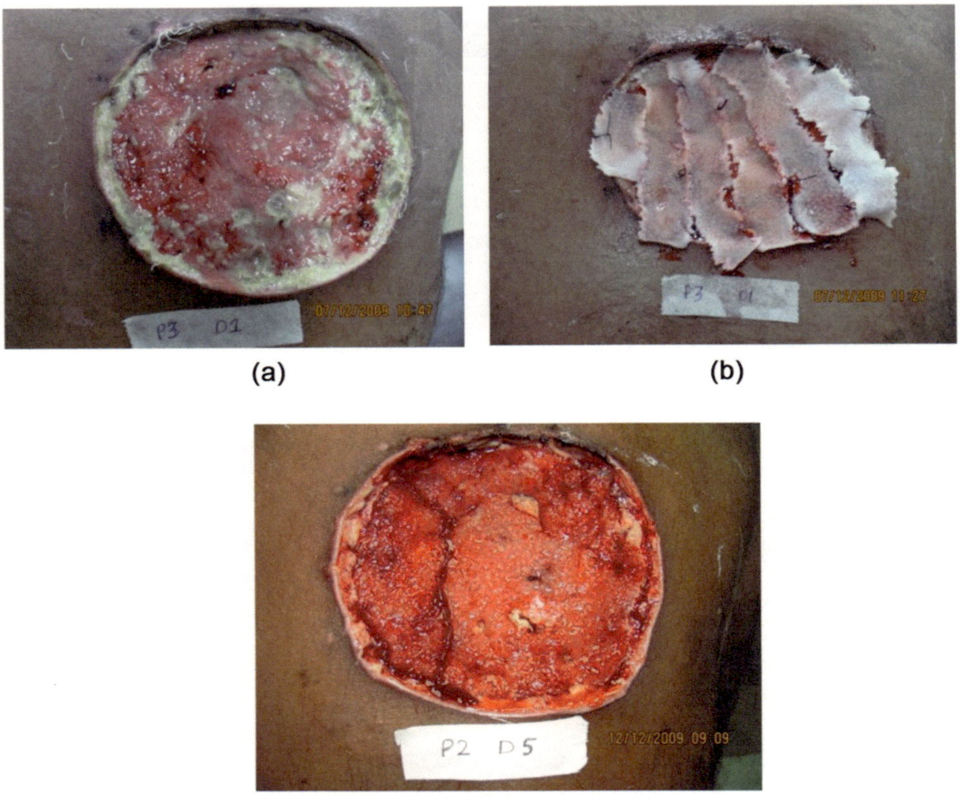

Figure 3.
a. Wound after excision of carbuncle. b. Application of porcine xenografts. c. Wound bed preparation on day 5.

Almost 40 years ago Ersek et al. [7] commented that porcine xenograft helps to maintain appropriate wound moisture and prevents cellular desiccation.

Though porcine xenograft was observed to be a useful temporary biological wound cover, it is not readily available in India. So, its use continues to require special efforts, and hence though feasible, it is not very common. This field is certainly open for a future venture in India.

4. Cadaveric skin allograft

Though the positive impact of cadaveric skin allografts has been well recognized for several decades, in India the first cadaver skin bank with the ability to procure, process, and store the allografts was established by the author and her supportive colleagues in April 2000 at LTM Medical College and General Hospital, Mumbai [8].

Burd [9] and others [10] associated mainly with burn management have noted that Allografts are more effective than Xenografts in achieving burn wound epithelization as well as wound bed preparation for subsequent wound closure with skin autograft. But the availability of cadaver skin allograft remains limited and hence alternative methods are essential.

The experience of the author in the utilization of skin allograft has been published [11] and is being shared here in brief with data updated to August 2010. Over about 10 years and 6 months cadaver skin allografts were used in 215 patients.

Indication	Number of patients (%)
Primary excision and temporary wound closure	56 (26.1%)
Promotion of epithelization	54 (25.1%)
Poor general condition	33 (15.3%)
Wound bed preparation	72 (33.5%)
Total	215 (100%)

Table 7.
Utilization of skin allografts.

The majority of these were burned patients except for seven patients (four with nonburn trauma and three with necrotizing fasciitis) in whom the allografts were used for wound bed preparation. The different clinical situations that led to the utilization of skin allografts have been shown in **Table 7**. The allografts provided remarkable pain relief besides promotion of epithelization reducing the need for autograft. Excellent wound bed preparation was achieved by control of infection (**Figure 4a–c**), maintenance of moisture balance, improved wound vascularization, and control of protein loss from wound leading to improved general condition. The autograft take was observed to be 100%. These effects have been observed by many [9, 12, 13]. Nonburn wounds too showed control of slough formation and improved vascularity with the use of skin allografts (**Figure 5a** and **b**). In case of failure of autograft take, use of skin allograft salvaged the situation and re grafting could be

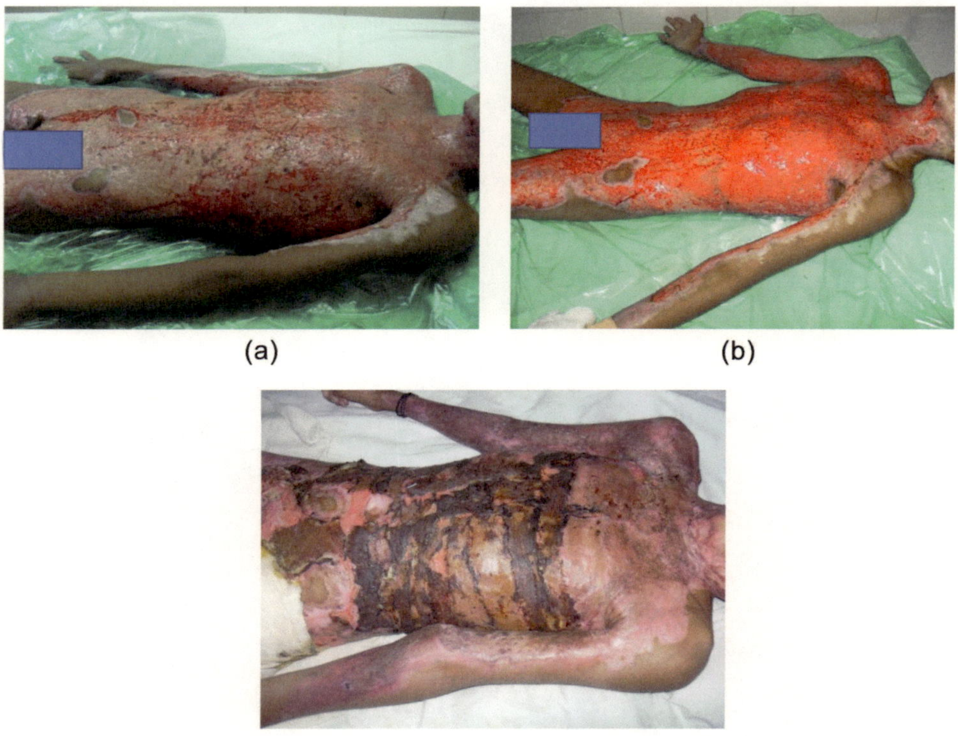

Figure 4.
a. Burn wound unsuitable for skin autograft due to infection, poor granulation. b. Wound bed preparation after application of skin allografts. c. Wound closure with autograft in two sittings.

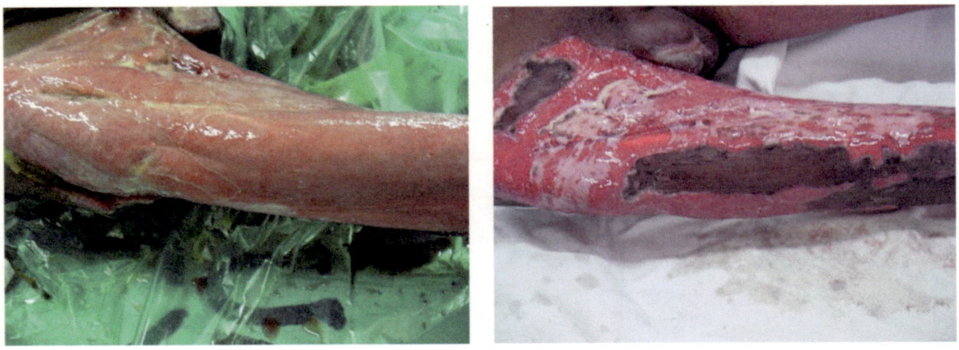

(a) (b)

Figure 5.
a. Necrotising fasciitis wound post debridement. b. Wound improvement with skin allografts.

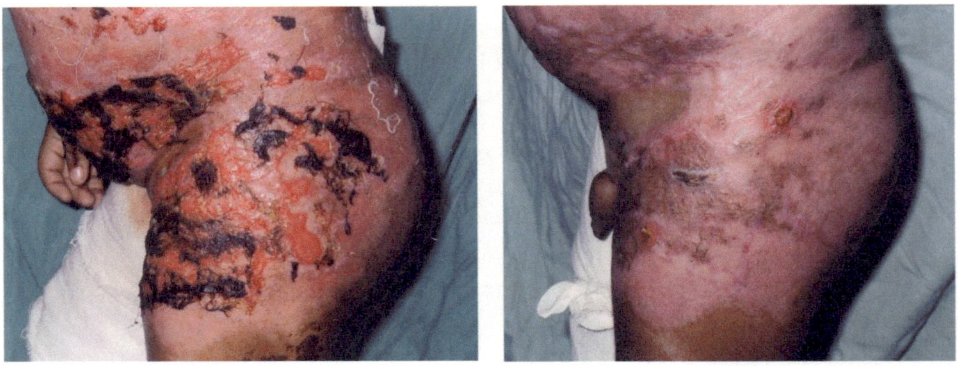

(a) (b)

Figure 6.
a. Loss of skin autograft. b. Salvage using skin allografts.

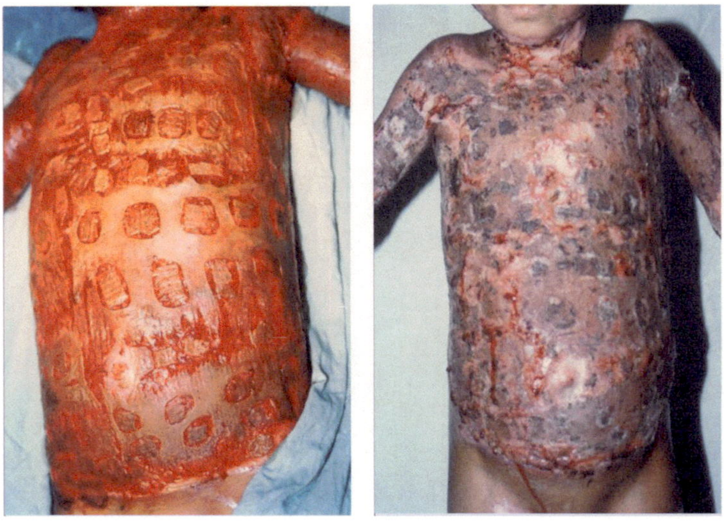

(a) (b)

Figure 7.
a. Intermingled skin allograft and autograft. b. Outcome of intermingled skin grafting.

avoided (**Figure 6a** and **b**). Allograft was used for wound closure as intermingled grafting (**Figure 7a** and **b**).

Skin allografts are also effective as method of temporary wound closure for chronic nonhealing wounds such as venous ulcers and diabetic ulcers as allografts stimulate the release of growth factors and cause modification of the wound micro-environment [14, 15].

4.1 Conclusion

Skin allograft was found to be extremely effective in controlling infection, improving wound vascularity, reducing pain, promoting epithelization, improving general condition—all this with fewer dressing change procedures. Once again it was apparent that skin alone is the best replacement for lost skin. But the possibility of disease transmission, the immunogenicity of allograft, and the limited availability of allografts are the main hurdles in the use of skin allografts. Probably, tissue-engineered skin would provide an effective but certainly expensive answer to achieve wound closure for many [13].

5. Barrier foam dressing

Several types of wound dressings are available and the choice depends on the condition of the wound. The condition of a wound may vary from time to time depending on multiple factors such as infection, slough, discharge, and hence the choice of appropriate dressing should also change accordingly. Moist wound healing is a well-accepted concept, but excessive wound exudate is harmful for optimal wound bed preparation as it damages the extracellular matrix. Foam is an absorptive material that can be useful as a dressing for exuding wounds [1]. Foams impregnated with antimicrobials (most often Silver) have been in use for more than a decade and these are drug-eluting type of dressings. The antimicrobial action of these agents needs penetration through the cell wall of the organism. This mechanism itself is likely to lead to the development of resistant organisms [16]. Besides, sustained release of antimicrobial is likely to lead to cytotoxicity.

To overcome this issue barrier foam dressing has been prepared using NIMBUS technology [17]. This has polyurethane foam coated with poly diallyl-dimethyl ammonium chloride which is a quaternary ammonium compound—a surface-active agent. The technology is such that it does not permit leaching of the active agent from the foam and the antimicrobial action is due to contact with the microbial cell wall and not by entry inside the organism. This mechanism prevents the development of resistant organisms [17]. The study conducted by Tran et al. revealed that this barrier foam dressing effectively inhibits bacterial attachment and the formation of biofilm [18]. The dressing can be used as primary dressing without the application additional topical agent on the wound.

An open-labeled study was conducted by the author to evaluate the safety and efficacy of barrier foam dressing. The study details and the outcome has been published [19].

5.1 Conclusion

On completion of the study, the conclusion was that the foam dressing was effective in absorbing and reducing the wound exudate which reflects control of wound infection (**Figure 8a** and **b**). It aided the separation of necrotic tissue from the wound bed and hence good wound bed preparation was achieved

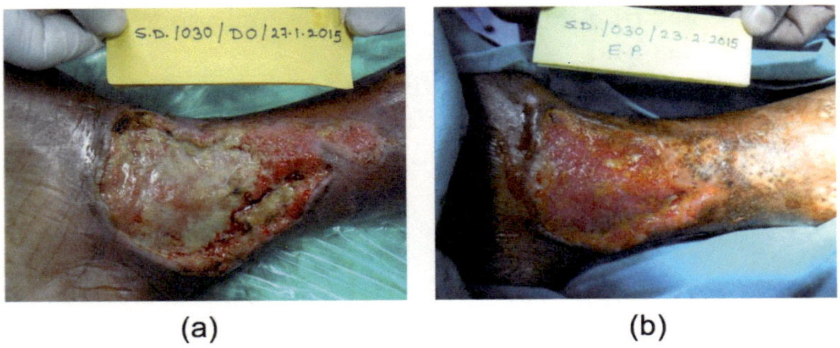

Figure 8.
a. Diabetic foot ulcer. b. Wound bed preparation at endpoint.

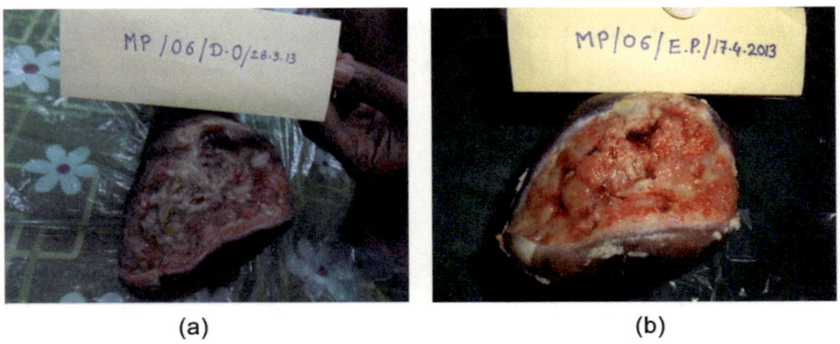

Figure 9.
a. Amputation stump. b. Wound bed preparation at endpoint.

(**Figure 9a** and **b**). Dressing change was not painful. It was easy to train the relatives to do the wound dressing.

This barrier foam dressing is now available commercially.

6. Discussion

From the moment a wound occurs its journey towards closure begins. Besides the management of systemic factors, the role played by different components of wound care methods is extremely crucial in augmenting the process of wound closure. The components include wound cleaning agents, methods of wound debridement, topical agents, various dressing materials, skin and skin substitutes, and specific methods such as Negative Pressure Wound Therapy (NPWT), multi-layered compression bandages. Some of these methods have been discussed in other chapters in this book.

Relatively simple modification like silver ion impregnation in porcine xenografts provides effective antimicrobial wound dressing for colonized chronic wounds according to Ersek [20]. This characteristic could be useful in wound bed preparation of significantly infected wounds with resistant organisms. A successful skin grafting procedure is life-saving for patients with large burns. Ersek has also reported significant improvement in the take of widely meshed skin autograft when covered with silver-impregnated porcine xenograft [21]. This modification would certainly increase the cost of the treatment but then our patient population does extend over a wide socioeconomic spectrum. The author has no personal experience of use of this product. New developments are always welcome but certainly, need appropriate evaluation and identification of indications for the use of new product or method.

DOI: http://dx.doi.org/10.5772/intechopen.102935

New technologies, new agents aiding debridement, new concepts related to temporary or permanent wound closure methods to aid wound bed preparation and wound closure will certainly continue to develop. Out of multiple methods available for wound bed preparation, the choice would continue to depend on the properties and quality of the method and the need of the wound at that point in time. The same method may not be appropriate for all wounds and hence thorough understanding of different methods is essential while working in the field of wound care. The choice of the method also depends on its availability, cost, affordability of the patient, access to the health care facility, the familiarity of the healthcare worker with the method, possible undesirable effects, and acceptance by the patient. Difficult access, financial constraints may make it necessary to train the family members of the patient to perform the wound care procedure. This situation would certainly have an impact on the choice of wound bed preparation method. Development of new methods will continue and consideration of all the above-mentioned issues is essential while conducting proper evaluation of these methods.

7. Conclusions

Here, the author has shared her experience of evaluating different methods from topical agent, barrier foam dressing to xenografts and allografts. Each of these has its place in wound bed preparation. The topical agent, indigenously prepared was found to be effective in controlling infection, inflammation and led to good wound bed preparation. But it is no longer available. The barrier foam dressing uses a different technology and was found suitable for infected, exuding wounds with necrotic material along with ease of dressing change and easy training of family members. Though the study was not a controlled trial, the author would prefer barrier foam dressing over the conventional wet to dry dressing method which is painful and training of family member is difficult. Porcine xenografts were found to be effective in control of infection, pain and aided epithelization and wound bed preparation leading to successful graft take. But consistent and focused effort is needed to make it available in India as an indigenous product. Skin allografts played an excellent role not only in preparing the wound bed, reducing the need for skin autograft but also lead to remarkable improvement in the general condition of the patient, particularly with large burn wounds. But deceased donor skin donation is still a relatively new concept in India, the availability of skin allograft is limited.

It is hoped that this sharing of experiences would provide food for thought, the stimulus for development of newer products using indigenously available resources, blooming of new concepts adaptable for the patient population in given region or country. The appropriate evaluation of these innovations would identify the indications, make them cost-effective and affordable to the vast population of patients with wounds spread all over the world.

Author details

Madhuri Gore
Zen Hospital, Mumbai, India

*Address all correspondence to: drmadhuri@hotmail.com

References

[1] Halim AS, Khoo TL, Mat Saad AZ. Wound bed preparation from a clinical perspective. Indian Journal of Plastic Surgery. 2012;**45**(2):193-202. DOI: 10.4103/0970-0358.101277

[2] Gore MA, Akolekar D. Evaluation of banana leaf dressing for partial thickness burn wounds. Burns. 2003;**29**(5):487-492. DOI: 10.1016/s0305-4179(03)00050-0

[3] Halim AS, Khoo TL, Yussof SJM. Biologic and synthetic skin substitutes: An overview. Indian Journal of Plastic Surgery. 2010;**43**(Suppl):S23-S28. DOI: 10.4103/0970-0358.70712

[4] Chiu T, Burd A. "Xenograft" dressing in the treatment of burns. Clinics in Dermatology. 2005;**23**(4):419-423. DOI: 10.1016/j.clindermatol.2004.07.027

[5] Bekeny JC, Kennedy C, Turissini JD, et al. Utility of porcine-derived xenograft as an adjunct to split-thickness skin grafting in lower-extremity wounds. Journal of the American Podiatric Medical Association. 2021;**111**(3):1-8. DOI: 10.7547/20-058

[6] Raimer DW, Group AR, Petitt MS, Nosrati N, et al. Porcine xenograft biosynthetic wound dressings for the management of Mohs wounds. Dermatology Online Journal. 2011;**17**(9):1. DOI: 10.5070/D37xp7m4cd

[7] Ersek RA, Hachen HJ. Porcine xenografts in the treatment of pressure ulcers. Annals of Plastic Surgery. 1980;**5**(6):464-470. DOI: 10.1097/00000637-198012000-00009

[8] Gore M. Cadaver skin donation and skin bank. Indian Journal of Burns. 2017;**25**(1):3. Available from: link.gale.com/apps/doc/A519525519/AONE?u=anon~ad9a29e5&sid=googleScholar&xid=d20993ee

[9] Burd A, Chiu T. Allogenic skin in the treatment of burns. Clinics in Dermatology. 2005;**23**(4):376-387. DOI: 10.1016/j.clindermatol.2004.07.019

[10] Wang H-J, Yeap CL, Heimbach DM. Allograft vs xenograft in preparation of wound for autograft. Journal of Burn Care and Rehabilitation. 1984;**5**(2):116-118. DOI: 10.1097/00004630-198403000-00006

[11] Gore MA, De AS. Deceased donor skin allograft banking: Response and utilization. Indian Journal of Plastic Surgery. 2010;**43**(Suppl):S114-S120. DOI: 10.4103/0970-0358.70732

[12] Imahara SD, Klein MB. Skin grafts. In: Orgill D, Blanco C, editors. Woodhead Publishing Series in Biomaterials, Biomaterials for Treating Skin Loss. Woodhead Publishing; 2009. pp. 58-79. ISBN: 9781845693633. DOI: 10.1533/9781845695545.1.58

[13] Sharma KS, Ralston D, Giblin V, MacNeil S. Engineering of accepted skin-equivalent tissue for tissue repair: Current state and perspectives. In: Reis RL, editor. Encyclopedia of Tissue Engineering and Regenerative Medicine. Academic Press; 2019. pp. 285-298. ISBN:9780128137000.DOI:10.1016/B978-0-12-801238-3.65568-X

[14] Snyder RJ. Treatment of nonhealing ulcers with allografts. Clinics in Dermatology. 2005;**23**(4):388-395. DOI: 10.1016/j.clindermatol.2004.07.020

[15] Kirsner RS, Margolis D, Masturzo A, et al. A real-world experience with the bioactive human split thickness skin allograft for venous leg ulcers; wound repair and regeneration. The International Journal of Tissue Repair and Regeneration. 2020;**28**(4):547-552

[16] Mikhaylova A, Liesenfeld B, Moore D, Toreki W, Vella J, et al.

Preclinical evaluation of antimicrobial efficacy and biocompatibility of a novel bacterial barrier dressing. Wounds. 2011;**23**(2):24-31

[17] Murata H, Koepsel RR, Matyjaszewski K, Russell AJ. Permanent, non-leaching antibacterial surface-2: How high density cationic surfaces kill bacterial cells. Biomaterials. 2007;**28**:4870-4879

[18] Tran PL, Hamood AN, De souza A, Schultz G, Liesenfeld B, et al. A study on the ability of quaternary ammonium groups attached to a polyurethane foam wound dressing to inhibit bacterial attachment and biofilm formation. Wound Repair and Regeneration. 2015;**23**:74-81. DOI: 10.1111/wrr.12244

[19] Gore M, Jadhav S, Schultz G, Mehta D. Evaluation of safety and efficacy of barrier foam dressing in patients with exuding wounds. Biomedical Journal of Scientific & Technical Research. 2021;**33**(5):26292-26297. ISSN: 2574-1241. DOI: 10.26717/BJSTR.2021.33.005475

[20] Ersek RA, Navarro JA. Maximizing wound healing with silver-impregnated porcine xenograft. Today's OR Nurse. 1990;**12**(12):4-9

[21] Ersek RA, Denton DR. Silver-impregnated porcine xenografts for treatment of meshed autografts. Annals of Plastic Surgery. 1984;**13**(6): 482-487. DOI: 10.1097/00000637-198412000-00004

Chapter 3

Haruan Extract (*Channa striatus*) as an Effective Mediator in Promoting Wound Healing

Ahmad Farouk Musa and Cheang Jia Min

Abstract

Wound healing remains a major issue in surgery. None of the existing treatment modalities in caring for wounds can yet claim to be the holy grail of wound management. *Channa striatus*, locally known in Malaysia as *Haruan*, is a freshwater air-breathing carnivorous fish that is proven to influence the different phases of wound healing. As a medicinal fish, not only does *Haruan* have a high content of amino and fatty acids, which are essential in collagen fibre synthesis during wound recovery, it also abounds in arachidonic acid and polyunsaturated fatty acids that promote prostaglandin synthesis, a vital component of the healing process. Moreover, its antinociceptive effects could potentially reduce wound pain, an important factor in wound healing. Proteomic studies show that a quarter of the total protein detected in freeze- and spray-dried *C. striatus* extract are actin, myosin and tropomyosin – all molecules that play a role in the wound healing process. Proteomic profiling also reveals that *Haruan* possesses two types of collagen namely collagen type-I and type-II that confer tensile strength during the healing process. It is proven that collagen along with other components of the extracellular matrix form the granulation tissue which, when contracted, closes the wound and concomitantly aligns the collagen fibres in the extracellular matrix. Hence, it is inferred that *Haruan* promotes the maturation of granulation tissue, thereby expediting the wound healing process itself. Consequently, it could mediate a faster recovery from surgical wound coupled with a lower incidence of wound infection due to an improved and accelerated wound healing process. Additionally, *Haruan* has demonstrated its ability in promoting angiogenesis and cell proliferation in wound bed preparation for skin grafting. Furthermore, a *Haruan* aerosol concentrate can act as a wound dressing at the donor site thereby enhancing the healing process while simultaneously exhibiting some antinociceptive properties. *Haruan*'s exceptional ability in promoting wound healing together with its potential use in skin grafting would be instrumental in the field of surgery. In essence, the cumulated benefits from all the processes involved would translate into a significant reduction of hospitalisation cost; that would immensely benefit not only the patient, but also the government.

Keywords: *Haruan*, *Channa striatus*, wound healing, proteomic studies, skin grafting, economic burden

1. Introduction

A wound is a mechanical injury to the body leading to disruption of the normal anatomical structure and function. It can be classified into acute and chronic wounds. Acute wounds normally proceed through the reparative process in an orderly and timely manner to restore anatomical and functional integrity. Conversely, wounds that demonstrate signs of delayed and interrupted healing and fail to go through the normal healing process are termed chronic wounds [1–3].

Wound healing reflects a cascade of complex, highly regulated biological events to restore the body's anatomical function back to its pre-injured state. Unlike acute wounds that heal by primary intention where the edges of the wound are apposed and held together with minimal scarring, chronic wounds heal by secondary intention [4, 5]; they form granulation tissue which fills the wound defects.

2. History of wound care and wound dressing

Wound management involves providing an optimum environment to promote healing, control bleeding and prevent infection. The history of wound care traces its origin to the Sumerians, a civilisation believed to be older than 2,000 BC [6]. In their manuscript, three healing gestures – cleansing the wounds, making the plasters and bandaging the wounds – were identified [7].

The ancient Egyptians and Greeks also contributed to the evolution of wound management. The Egyptian medical papyri documented the principle of wound closure to aid healing and the utilisation of honey, grease and lint as the main constituents of the most common plaster. It was believed that lint, a derivative of vegetable fibre, serves an absorbent role; grease or animal fat forms a barrier against bacteria; and honey, the most frequently cited ingredient in multiple topical wound preparations, possesses various healing and antibacterial properties favourable for wound healing [8, 9].

Interestingly, the Greeks were the first to recognise the difference between infected and uninfected wounds, using terms such as "fresh" or "non-healing" to describe wounds [10, 11]. Galen of Pergamum (120–201 AD) is a Greek surgeon who made remarkable contributions to wound and haemorrhage management. He emphasised the maintenance of wound moisture and the application of styptics consisting of basic elements with antibiotic properties for optimum wound healing [12, 13]. Despite advances in modern technology, Galen's basic principles are still incorporated into the development of current wound dressings.

Additionally, the Hippocratic collection discussed the addition of wine to obstinate ulcer for maximal wound healing [13]. Indeed, in ancient times, a number of magical and mythological agents were utilised as wound dressings; they include honey, plaster, wine and milk. While some of them demonstrate significant pharmacological roles, others merely have ritualistic meanings [13].

In the modern era, a wide array of dressings and wound care products with their properties tailored to special wound care needs were invented. In fact, Winter's study [10–13], which concluded that moisturised wounds heal quicker than dry wounds, sparked an explosive burst in the evolution of wound dressings. Thanks to modern technology, novel techniques such as the adoption of growth factors, bioengineered tissue, negative pressure therapy and hyperbaric oxygen therapy are nowadays implemented in wound management. Nonetheless, none of the existing modalities can claim to be the holy grail of wound management.

Alongside the cosmetic advancement in the past decades, skin grafting – a source of epithelium for both acute and chronic wounds – has become increasingly prevalent [14, 15]. However, quite surprisingly, skin grafting is not a new concept; for the past 3500 years, it has been extensively practised by a string of renowned physicians. These include Aulus Cornelius Celsus (25 BC - 50 AD), the Roman author of the first systematic treatise on Medicine; Claudius Gelenus (129 AD - 210 AD) popularly known as Galen, a prominent Greek physician; Jaques-Louis Reverdin (1842–1929), the Swiss surgeon who performed the first "fresh skin" allograft; and George David Pollock (1817–1897), a British surgeon known as a pioneer of skin grafts [16–24]. Throughout the years, the roles and functions of skin grafting have expanded. Nowadays, skin graft is an indispensable therapy in burn reconstruction, major traumatic injuries and surgical defects [25, 26]. Nonetheless, it still suffers from major drawbacks such as compromised skin grafts, skin graft rejection and skin graft contractions particularly in elderly patients, immunocompromised individuals and those on immunosuppressant medications [27–35].

Meanwhile, TIME – a concept that stands for Tissue, Infection or Inflammation, Moisture, and Epithelial edge advancement – is a new framework of wound bed preparation initiated by Schultz and his team in 2003 to achieve optimal wound healing [36, 37]. As the freshwater fish *Haruan* is naturally gifted with numerous antinociceptive and antimicrobial capabilities, high water content and ample amounts of amino acids and polyunsaturated fatty acids essential for granulation tissues formation and epithelialisation, it fits the components of Tissue, Infection and Moisture in the TIME framework. Therefore, we can postulate that *Haruan* fish also has the potential to function as an effective wound dressing.

3. Stages of wound healing

The phases of wound healing is a continuum that encompasses homeostasis, inflammatory, proliferative and maturation phases under stringent regulation of growth factors, cytokines, and chemokines [38]. Admittedly, the various phases of the wound healing process can overlap and go awry anytime. The inflammatory phase is the shortest of all phases and, if arrested, wound healing will be delayed and fibrosed tissue may be formed. Meanwhile, in the proliferative phase, the wound is shrunken in size until the maturation phase. Despite the surface of the wounds being closed completely, full tensile strength might take up to twelve months to develop [3, 4, 38–40]. **Table 1** below describes the different stages, mechanisms and molecules at interplay during the wound healing process.

Unfortunately, despite the enormous efforts made in skin repair, a wound can never achieve the maximum tensile strength of a normal skin. Additionally, owing to its tight regulation by a multitude of factors, proper wound healing can be easily impeded. Indeed, chronic non-healing wounds are a common phenomenon. **Figure 1** describes both the intrinsic and extrinsic factors that affect wound healing.

Stages	Mechanism	Main molecules
Homeostasis	• Vasoconstriction • Initiation of coagulation cascade • Formation of clot at the site of injury	• Complement prostaglandins • Vascular endothelial transforming growth factors • Nitric oxide • Cytokines • Platelets
Inflammatory	• Vasodilatation • Recruit and activation of neutrophils and macrophages for phagocytosis • Synthesis of wound exudate	• Cytokines • Growth factors • Neutrophils • Monocytes and macrophages
Proliferative	• Formation and proliferation of granulation tissues • Fibroblasts and collagen production • Formation of vascular network via angiogenesis • Contraction – contractile cells pull the wound margins together • Epithelialisation – growth of epidermal cells over the surface of the granulation tissue	• Fibroblasts • Macrophages • Collagen • Extracellular ground substance • Growth factors • Proteases • Epidermal cells
Maturation	• Fibroblasts reduce in number • Vascularisation decreases • Tensile strength increases	• Fibroblasts • Collagen • Matrix metalloproteinases (MMPs) and inhibitors

Table 1.
Stages of wound healing [3, 4, 38–40].

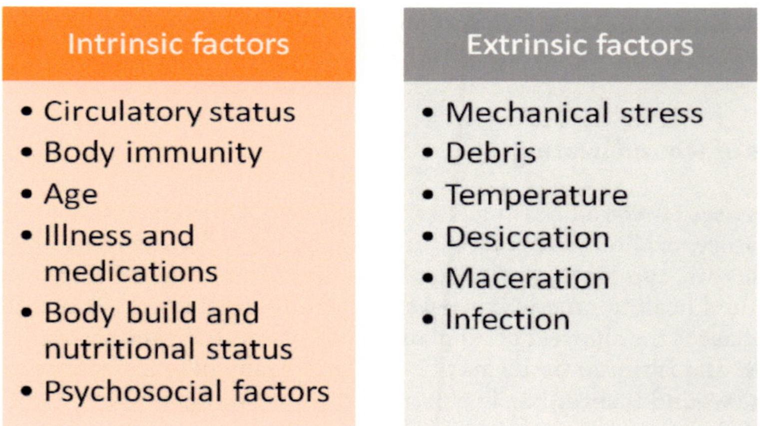

Figure 1.
Factors that affect wound healing.

4. What is *Haruan*

Channa striatus or snakehead murrel, commonly known as *Haruan* or *Gabus* in the Southeast Asian region, originates from the family *Channidae* or *Ophiocephalidae* [41]. It is a tropical, aerobic, carnivorous freshwater species measuring around 100 cm. It is sexually active at 30 cm, with a dark dorsal surface and sides, and mottled with a combination of black and ochre; it also has a white belly, a large head resembling a snake and a fully-toothed mouth with large scales. It preys on smaller fishes and frogs for survival. Since *C. striatus* is an obligate air-breather, it survives by burrowing in muds of lakes, rivers or canals, keeping its skin and air-breathing apparatus moist while surviving on stored fats [42, 43]. Wild *Haruan* lives a solitary life except in the spawning season. **Figure 2** shows a solitary *Haruan* in an aquarium with a glass reflection showing its white belly.

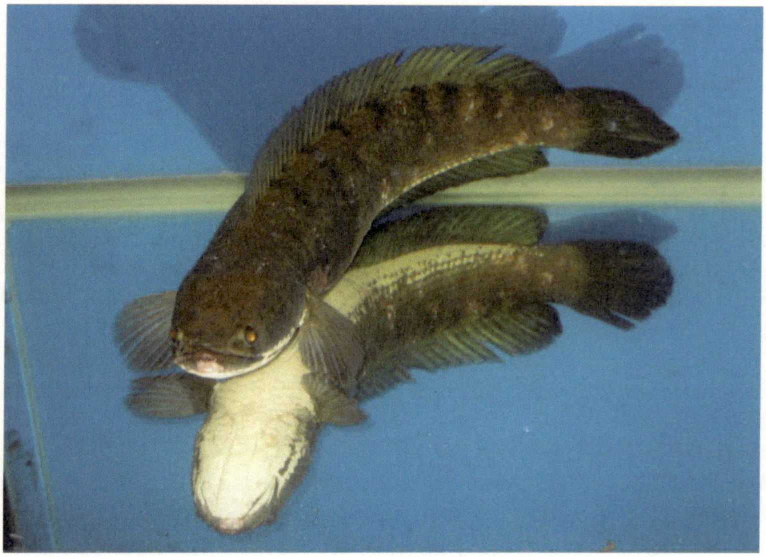

Figure 2.
Wild Haruan - Channa striatus - in an aquarium.

Pairs breed during most months of the year, laying hundreds of amber-coloured eggs. The eggs, guarded by both parents, are non-adhesive and they hatch within one to three days. The adults have compact muscles and a less bony structure which give them the desirable characteristics of a predatory fish [43]. Besides, they are highly aggressive predators with the ability to travel overland to exploit new bodies of water [42]. **Figure 3** describes the characteristics of *Channa striatus* or *Haruan*.

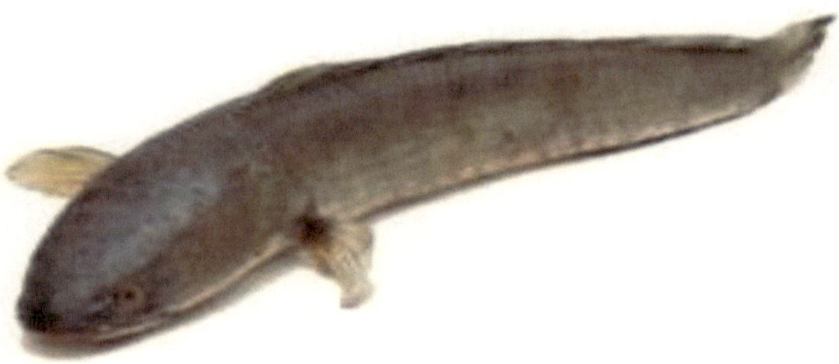

Figure 3.
Summary of the characteristics of Haruan species [41–43].

- Obligate air-breathing species
- Cavernous freshwater fish
- Common habitats: small ditches, ponds, rivers, lakes, rice fields
- Ideal water temperature for survival: around 20–30°C
- Depth of water: below two meters
- pH of habitat: 4.30 to 7.90

Haruan fish can be farmed though it is considered a pest or predatory species in Europe, North America and Australia, being a voracious predator and a competitor of native fish species [44, 45]. When it is reared in a controlled habitat, the parameters of the aquatic environment such as the pH, temperature and water depth should be kept as close to its natural habitat as possible. For its diet, *Haruan* fish can be fed with a wide range of food products including formulated food [46–48].

However, compared to other species such as *Keli* or *Tilapia* fish, *Haruan* fish farming is not popular for two reasons: firstly, being a predator, it can easily eat up the surrounding aquatic animals and small terrestrial rodents; secondly, its commercial benefits have not been extensively publicised to receive enough attention [49, 50].

In Malaysia, *Haruan* fish is cherished as a wholesome delicacy; it is served in a multitude of preparations ranging from steamed, grilled, spiced, fried, roasted, in the form of soup to even raw [51]. According to a study [52] conducted by Haemamalar and his team in Krau Wildlife Reserve, *Haruan* fish was reported to be one of the sources of freshwater fish among the Orang Asli (aboriginal people) tribunates.

Additionally, *Haruan* serves as a natural remedy for the local population. The National Health and Morbidity Survey carried out in 2014 [53], which looked at the prevalence of food supplements and the reasons for their intake, demonstrated that of the 0.68% of Malaysians consuming *Haruan* as a dietary supplement, 90.82% did so based on its alleged health benefits.

Thanks to the Chinese and Malay communities, *Haruan* has acquired a reputation for wound healing for the past several decades [54]. Poh *et al* did a research [55] involving a total of 134 Chinese mothers during the months of childbirth; they found out that *Haruan* fish was reported by a quarter of the participating women as either a necessary or a recommended food owing to its wound healing property [56]. Nonetheless, the wound healing effect of *Haruan* was merely anecdotal until two recently published clinical trials [57, 58] scientifically confirmed this common belief.

5. Preparation of *Haruan*

5.1 Cooking

Different cooking methods of *Haruan* fish can generate different outcomes. For instance, *Haruan* fish fillets preserve their nutritional value when grilled but absorb too much oil when fried, which can be detrimental to health [59]. Meanwhile, when prepared in soup, the time and heat utilised have to be properly adjusted for the snakehead fish to retain its nutritional value [60].

5.2 Topical agent

Haruan fish can also be converted into a topical agent in the form of spray or cream. This preparation involves the addition of a propellant (spray) or aqua cream (cream) to the *Haruan* extract [61, 62]. When *Haruan* is formulated into aerosol concentrate and sprayed on a wound, it will form a thin layer of dressing that acts as a protective barrier against the outside environment [63]. This minimises the physical pain as well as the mental suffering associated with dressing application and removal [64].

5.3 Haruan capsules

The principal author of this chapter worked collaboratively with the School of Pharmacy, Universiti Sains Malaysia, to process *Haruan* capsules for his research work together with fellow surgeons at the National Heart Institute, Kuala Lumpur, several years ago. Admittedly, oral *Haruan* supplement has a higher amount of concentrate which is believed to yield more merits compared to eating the flesh itself. Besides, for surgical or major traumatic wounds that involve multiple tissue layers, oral administration of *Haruan* extract is deemed superior to topical application [65, 66]. The detailed steps in the preparation of *Haruan* capsules are described in **Figure 4**.

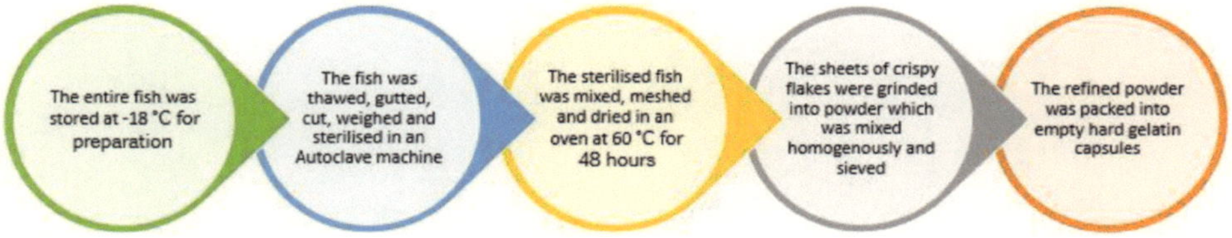

Figure 4.
Preparation of Haruan capsules [57].

6. Laboratory works

6.1 Chemical properties

Haruan is considered a crucial source of protein (78.32 ± 0.23%), lipid (2.08 ± 0.08%) and vitamin A (0.265 ± 0.013 mg) [49, 67, 68]. A proximate analysis of *Haruan* revealed that the ratio of crude protein, crude fat to crude ash in *Haruan* is 23:5.7:1.8 [67, 68]. In fact, *Haruan* is rich in amino acids and fatty acids, particularly glycine and arginine, which help minimise protein losses and enhance collagen synthesis essential for wound healing [56, 69, 70].

Interestingly, *Haruan* also synthesises polyunsaturated fatty acids, which accelerate wound healing via the mediation of prostaglandin and thromboxane synthesis [49, 68, 71–73]. Furthermore, apart from the major fatty acids such as stearic acid and linoleic acid [56, 74], *Haruan* possesses an unusually high profile of arachidonic acid (AA) and docosahexaenoic acid (DHA) which lower the risk of coronary artery disease [56, 67, 68, 75–77]. In terms of dietary nutritional elements, micronutrients such as magnesium, copper, zinc, iron, calcium and manganese and trace amounts of nickel and lead are also present in *Haruan* [78–80].

6.2 Antimicrobial effects

Exposed to an aquatic environment full of microbiota, fish usually develop their own immunity to safeguard against pathogens [81–83]. As a front-liner and paramount component of the innate immune system, fish mucus possesses a broad array of proteins and enzymes such as lysozyme, immunoglobulin, complement proteins, lectins and proteolytic enzymes that can phagocytose and digest micro-organisms [84–90]. Furthermore, it constantly secretes and sloughs off the skin to avoid adherence and prolonged colonisation by parasites [84–89]. Hence, fish skin mucus is regarded as a potential antibacterial therapeutic agent [91, 92]. The multiple roles of *Haruan* mucus are described in **Figure 5**.

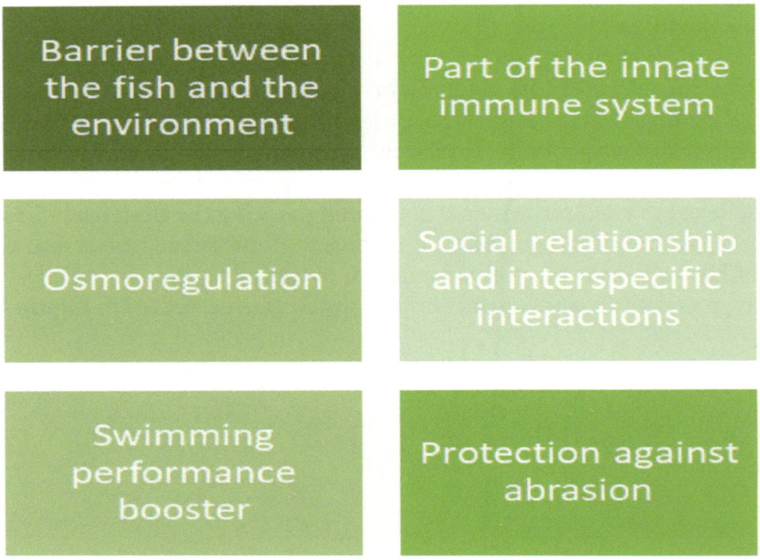

Figure 5.
Roles of the fish mucus [91, 92].

In recent years, extensive work has been conducted to analyse the antibacterial effects of the mucus of fish species [93–97], including the *Channa* species. Several research studies [48, 98–104] were performed over the years to evaluate the antibacterial and antifungal activities of *Haruan*. Most of the studies [99–104] revealed that *Haruan* displays some antimicrobial activities, except two studies [98, 99] which detected negligible inhibitory effects against *Staphylococcus aureus* and *Escherichia coli* strains respectively. As wound infection and dehiscence – two disastrous yet frequent complications of surgical wounds – are the common factors of delayed wound healing, the antimicrobial activity of *Haruan* is an added merit for wound dressing [105–107].

6.3 Antinociceptive properties

Pain can have a deleterious impact on wound healing [108, 109]. Coupled with chronic inflammation, prolonged pain can trigger a vicious cycle that hinders wound healing [110]. Fortunately, appropriate wound dressings with sufficient pain control can enormously improve wound healing outcomes, with accelerated wound healing and, consequently, a shorter hospital stay [111].

The antinociceptive effects of *Haruan* in postoperative and traumatic patients have long been discussed and reported. For instance, an earlier *Haruan* study [112] conducted abdominal constriction and tail flick test on mice and found that *Haruan* not only possesses peripherally-acting antinociceptive activity, but its extracts could also act synergistically with other painkillers such as morphine to relieve postoperative pain and discomfort. These findings are supported by another study conducted by Solihah *et al* [113] who presented a similar positive result. The underlying mechanism is thought to be attributed to the presence of fatty acids and amino acids, particularly arginine, glycine and arachidonic acid, in addition to the involvement of the L-arginine-nitric oxide-cGMP pathway [42, 114]. In fact, the antinociceptive effects *Haruan* remain relatively stable in a wide range of temperature and pH; this allows the essence to be extracted and processed safely for future use [115].

6.4 Wound healing capabilities

Freshwater fish constitute 60–70% of the animal protein intake in Malaysia [116]. Previous studies demonstrated that *Haruan* contains a high content of albumin which promotes the formation of collagen [117–119]. Moreover, it has a considerable amount of copper and zinc that can help accelerate wound healing by maintaining cell stability, besides promoting wound remodelling and the formation of blood vessels and fibrosis or scar [119–124]. Additionally, the presence of elements such as hydroxyproline, glycine, arachidonic acid and arginine in *Haruan* is another essential source of collagen [124–126].

It is therefore no surprise that the collagen content in *Haruan* is relatively high. Indeed, collagen plays a determining role in expediting wound healing via various mechanisms. According to Kwan *et al* who performed proteometric profiling of *Haruan*, two types of collagen, namely type I and type II collagen, were detected [127, 128]. Both of them increase the tensile strength [129]. In fact, when the increased tensile strength and glycosaminoglycan of *Haruan* was examined and compared to cetrimide, it was reported that *Haruan* is superior to cetrimide in improving wound contraction and the fibroblastic phase of wound healing [61, 130, 131]. Furthermore, it was found that the collagen in *Haruan* can help promote the maturation of granulation tissue which accelerates wound healing. *Haruan* can act in synchrony with the other components of the extracellular matrix to form a granulation tissue which subsequently contracts and seals the wound. Concurrently, it aligns the collagen fibres in the extracellular matrix. If the area of involvement is wide enough, the granulation tissue could be reserved for split skin grafting. The various steps of collagen involvement in wound healing are described in **Figure 6**.

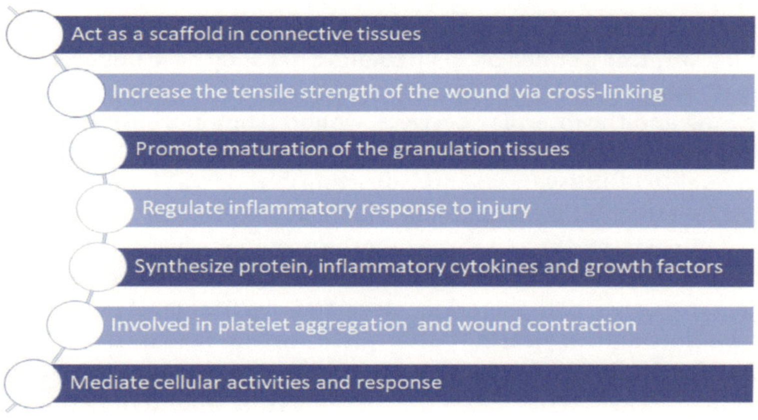

Figure 6.
Wound healing effects of collagen [132–135].

According to the researchers [128] who performed proteomic profiling of *Haruan* extract at the Analytical Biochemistry Research Centre, Universiti Sains Malaysia, the proportion of actin, myosin and tropomyosin to the total protein in freeze-dried and spray-dried *Haruan* water extract are 25% and 26% respectively. While it is known that these three structures play a significant role in muscle contraction in the sliding filament theory, many were unaware that that they also work hand-in-hand in the wound healing process. Tropomyosin can help control cell functioning of actin while actin can regulate vital cellular functions during re-epithelisation involving cell division, cytokinesis and cell signalling, seal the embryonic wound as well as interact with myosin in the regulation of cell motility [132–134]. The functions of actin, myosin, and tropomyosin during the wound healing process are diagrammatically summarised in **Figure 7**.

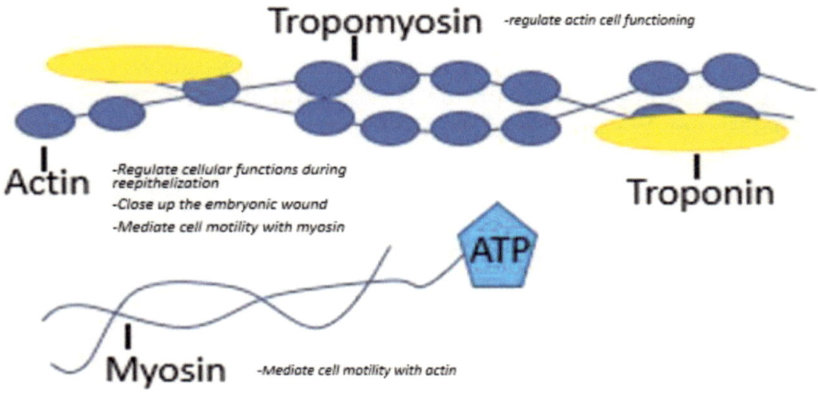

Figure 7.
Functions of actin, myosin, and tropomyosin in wound healing [57, 128].

7. Clinical trials on *Haruan*

To the best of our knowledge, only two clinical trials have reported the effects of *Haruan* in wound healing to date.

One study [57] was conducted by the principal author of this chapter. The researchers performed a double-blinded, randomised, controlled trial in 2018 at the National Heart Institute to look at the effects of *Haruan* fish extracts on the chest and leg surgical wounds of 253 patients after they have undergone coronary artery bypass surgery (CABG). Noting the detrimental impact of wound pain on wound healing and the interplay between wound pain, morbidity, quality of life and hospital stay [135–137], parameters such as wound pain and healing, mobilisation and quality of life were specifically evaluated. It was found that the wound scoring system favoured those patients who received *Haruan* capsules instead of placebo at day-6, six-weeks and three months postoperatively. They also discovered that *Haruan* extracts could alleviate wound pain, and improve quality of life with respect to energy, pain, emotion, sleep and physical level except social level based on the Nottingham Health Profile questionnaire that assesses the quality of life [57]. Therefore, *Haruan* extract is considered a cost-effective solution in wound healing because it decreases the percentage of wound infection thereby reducing the cost of hospitalisation. Moreover, with the patient's surgical recovery hastened, it can tremendously reduce the economic burden not only to the hospital but to the country as well.

Meanwhile, a similar study [58] conducted by Wahab *et al* targeted 76 post-lower segment Caesarean Section women, a study population which are the dominant consumers of *Haruan* in Malaysia due to old beliefs and food taboos [55, 56]. The study concluded that *Haruan* could improve the wound's cosmetic appearance and, accordingly, patient's satisfaction. These findings are in line with a randomised controlled trial [138] which reported that *Haruan* extract consumers harboured a remarkably higher rate of uterine involution than the placebo group. Conversely, in the same study, the outcomes of wound healing and pain were noted to be comparable; this can be attributed to the interval used for the pain score assessment and the concomitant use of analgesics.

8. Potential role of *Haruan* in skin grafting

Skin grafting is the transfer of cutaneous tissue to cover large wounds. It can take two forms: split skin grafting, which involves the epidermis and a portion of the dermis, and full-thickness skin grafting which involves the epidermis and the entire dermis [139]. While deliberating on the pros and cons of split skin grafting as compared to full thickness skin grafting is beyond the scope of this paper, it is noteworthy that a split skin graft does not have its own blood supply; it relies on the wound bed. This is where *Haruan* might play an important role. In their seminal work on the bioactive proteins in *C. striatus*, Kwan *et al* [140] have shown that the fish proteins promote angiogenesis and cell proliferation. The stable, healthy and well-vascularised wound bed potentiated by *Haruan* action allows for skin grafts to be well taken.

The main challenge to ensure that *Haruan* play its magical role in promoting angiogenesis and cell proliferation lies in the wound bed preparation before skin grafting. To ensure that the wound bed is healthy, wound debridement is of utmost importance. This could be done in several ways: via a scalpel, a dermatome, or even by using a hydro-surgery device until the wound bed is really clean and healthy with some bleeding at the wound bed [141]. It has to be stressed here that without a clean and healthy wound bed, and wound edges cleared from any necrotic or purulent tissue, the added value of *Haruan* would be lost and the skin graft will not have a proper healing.

When the wound bed is well prepared, skin grafts will normally go through three different stages as follows:

a. Imbibition: Oxygen and nutrients from the wound bed are passively absorbed by the skin graft [142].

b. Inosculation: A vascular connection is established between the cut vessels on the underside of the skin graft and the wound bed [143].

c. Revascularisation: Neoangiogenesis or new blood vessels grow into the graft from the wound bed [144].

After undergoing these stages, the skin grafts will usually need another five to seven days to adhere to the wound bed followed by the process of maturation that could last from several months to years; this includes pigmentation changes, softening and flattening [139]. As described earlier, *Haruan* abounds in amino acids in such as glycine, lysine and arginine, and fatty acids such as arachidonic acid, palmitic acid and docosahexaenoic acid – they all help to enhance wound healing through the initiation of several pathways including the remodelling of collagen that gives the strength to the wound, besides stimulating wound contraction [145].

Having discussed at length regarding the recipient site, we should also look at whether *Haruan* plays any role in wound healing at the donor site. Theoretically, the donor site requires wound care only in terms of wound dressing. Since the wound edges are not approximated at the donor site and are left to heal via secondary intention, they will be filled by granulation tissue matrix [146] and can be covered by a simple dressing only. Presumably this is another area in skin grafting where *Haruan* dressing might play a role. An aerosol concentrate containing *Haruan* water extract was formulated in an aerosol system to produce a thin film over the wound bed and serve as a dressing at the donor site [147]. The aerosol concentrate that would form a thin layer of dressing over the wound could enhance the healing process at the donor site as proven in an animal model [148], besides showing pronounced antinociceptive properties [149].

9. Other usages of *Haruan*

Apart from its aforementioned desirable features, *Haruan* has also been reported to confer feasible outcomes in a myriad of diseases.

Osteoarthritis is a degenerative joint disease characterised by synovial inflammation and articular cartilage degradation that leads to chronic pain and inflammation [150, 151]. In osteoarthritis, a wide variety of inflammatory mediators are secreted and activated [140]. After several previous studies which demonstrated the anti-inflammatory capabilities of *Haruan*, the role of *Haruan* in osteoarthritis has been extensively explored [152–154]. Few scientific reports on the efficacy of *Haruan* in osteoarthritic patients revealed promising outcomes where *Haruan* was shown to be superior in reducing inflammatory changes in the synovial membrane, improving the pain, symptoms and quality of life of osteoarthritic sufferers while maintaining the structure of the cartilage of the control group [155–159]. As osteoarthritis is a common complication of major traumatic wound injury, which necessitates skin grafting owing to the disfigurement and disabling condition, oral administration of *Haruan* can exert a double action, improving both wound healing and osteoarthritis.

Other functions of *Haruan* mentioned in the medical literature include its usage in allergic rhinitis [160, 161], dermatitis [162, 163], gastric ulcer [164, 165], cancer [166, 167], hypertension [168, 169] and depression [170, 171]. Unfortunately, due to the paucity of studies to date, further high-powered studies are warranted to clarify and define the role of *Haruan* in these diseases.

10. Discussion

Hong *et al* [65] did a scoping review on the effectiveness of *Haruan* extracts on wound healing; they concluded that current evidence favours the use of *Haruan* extracts to expedite wound healing. Indeed, optimal wound bed preparation and proper wound closure are the two fundamental goals of skin grafting regardless of the graft type [172–174]. With its extraordinary antimicrobial, antinociceptive and anti-inflammatory properties, *Haruan* is undeniably a handy tool for skin grafting. From a psychological perspective, *Haruan* can minimise post-operative pain and discomfort, achieve satisfactory aesthetic wound effect and improve patient postoperative quality of life. For skin grafting that covers a wound area only partially, *Haruan* can promote wound closure since it encourages the epithelialisation of wound. When a wound recovery is sped up with less wound infection, the duration of hospital stay will also be shortened. Consequently, expenses related to skin grafting will be cut down.

It is still inconclusive which particular biomolecules play a role in the wound healing property. However, with the advancement of technology especially in the field of proteomics, we have managed to conduct a more comprehensive protein profiling [175, 176]. Although proteomics helps us to understand the interactions between the proteins in the fish and the wound, the previous protein profiling [177] were not as accurate as the new one due to the lower sensitivity of the old equipment. Conversely, the current work using Gel Elution Liquid Fractionation Entrapment Electrophoresis (GELFREE) system can maximise protein profiling [127]. The researchers at the Analytical Biochemistry Research Centre of the Universiti Sains Malaysia [127, 128] also looked at the post-translational modifications (PTMs) of proteins which might be involved in the wound healing process to complement the protein profiling results. PTMs, as the name suggests, occurs following the translation of amino acids in the later part of the protein biosynthesis. They play an important role in protein regulation and are also involved in the regulation of a number of physiological functions. This helps us to appreciate how the consumption of *Haruan* contributes to the wound healing mechanism.

It is a known fact that structural proteins such as actin, myosin and tropomyosin are vital in the formation of muscle tissue within an organism. From the protein profiling, it was shown that 37% of all the proteins detected in the fish meat are structural proteins which play a specific role in enhancing wound healing. For example, actin gives rise to the formation of myofibroblasts which differentiated from fibroblasts containing bundles of actin microfilaments with contractile proteins such as non-muscle myosin [178–180]. On the one hand, both fibroblasts and myofibroblasts regulate traction force and coordinate contraction during wound closure [181]. On the other hand, tropomyosin, has been reported to regulate cell migration, particularly fibroblast and myofibroblasts [182]. This results in the promotion of rapid wound healing whenever tropomyosin is manipulated in the wound area [183, 184]. Hence, the abundant presence of structural proteins in the fish meat could be a key reason why it helps in the wound healing process.

Apart from structural proteins, *Haruan* meat also possesses numerous enzymes including trypsin. Trypsin has been shown to enhance the healing process by potentiating fibrocyte differentiation [185]. Trypsin has also been used as a biomedicine for treating wound [186]. A clinical study conducted by Gudmunssdsdóttir *et al* [175] showed that native-proteins were digested by cold-adapted cod trypsin and produced an encouraging effect on the wound. These findings supported the idea that the abundant level of trypsin in *Haruan* meat helps in facilitating the wound healing process.

Collagen, which is essential for wound healing, is also present in the *Channa striatus* meat with Collagen Type-I being the most abundant [127]. Collagen is required in the different stages of wound healing including the binding process to fibronectin that helps in platelet aggregation [187], triggering angiogenesis by transforming myocytes into macrophages [188], in addition to giving support to budding capillaries [189]. A recent study by Helary *et al* [190] has also shown that apoptosis was prevented during chronic wound treatment by the use of concentrated collagen hydrogel that promotes cell proliferation and protects fibroblasts. Recently, mammalian collagen has been replaced by fish collagen [191] which is considered a regenerative medicine [192], a sign that the abundant collagen found in fish meat does help to advance the wound healing process.

Results from the proteomic study [127] also show that *C. striatus* meat is rich in calcium related proteins such as calmodulin and parvalbumin. We are aware that calcium (Ca^{2+}) plays a major role in maintaining homeostasis of the skin and is considered a key signalling molecule during wound healing [193, 194]. Ca^{2+} binding proteins are also known to assist in Ca^{2+} signalling and skin intracellular trafficking, which includes calmodulin and calmodulin-like proteins [195]. It is also known that

Calmodulin assists in keratinocytes maturation [196], proving its significant role in the wound healing process. The important role played by both calmodulin and parvalbumin in the wound healing cascade deserves to be highlighted. Expression of parvalbumin in ependymal cells has been shown to assist in tissue remodelling and wound closure [197]. Hence, it is clear that both parvalbumin and calmodulin help to transfer Ca2+ to the affected area, thereby promoting wound healing.

Proteomic profiling also revealed that more than 50% of the total proteins detected in *C. striatus* are uncharacterised proteins [128]. The functions of these proteins are still unknown due to the paucity of research. These proteins have been labelled as such due to the absence of any detectable homology to those proteins of known functions at both the sequence and structural level [198]. However, it is possible that one or more of the uncharacterised proteins found in *Haruan* play a role in the wound healing process. Indeed, the high quantity of uncharacterised proteins detected via proteomics, that is, the proteome database for *C. striatus*, is far from complete. At this point in time, we can safely say that while existing data have given us an insight into the proteins of *Haruan,* more rigorous effort must be made into the research of the uncharacterised proteins that might be involved in accelerating the wound healing process – the indisputable characteristic of *C. striatus* or *Haruan.*

11. Conclusion

As a wound cosmetic enhancer as well as an antimicrobial, anti-inflammatory and antinociceptive agent, *Haruan* fish is a promising medicinal food product for wound healing. Current evidence has illustrated the effectiveness of *Haruan* in wound healing, particularly in postoperative patients. This book chapter has highlighted the wonders of *Haruan* in wound healing associated with skin grafting. Unfortunately, in spite of the emerging role and increasing popularity of *Haruan* in wound healing, the use of *Haruan* extracts in skin grafting remains insufficient. When its merits have been fully explored, *Haruan* extracts could become a viable alternative to the current wound dressing regimen in skin grafting in the near future.

Acknowledgements

The authors would like to express their gratitude to Nageeb Gounjaria for proofreading and editing the manuscript.

Author details

Ahmad Farouk Musa* and Cheang Jia Min
Jeffrey Cheah School of Medicine and Health Sciences, Monash University Malaysia, Malaysia

*Address all correspondence to: farouk@monash.edu

References

[1] Lazarus GS, Cooper DM, Knighton DR, Margolis DJ, Percoraro RE, Rodeheaver G, Robson MC. Definitions and guidelines for assessment of wounds and evaluation of healing. Wound repair and regeneration. 1994; 2(3):165-70.

[2] Swanson T, Keast D, Cooper R, Black J, Angel D, Schultz G, Carville K, Fletcher J. Ten top tips: identification of wound infection in a chronic wound. Wounds International. 2015; 6(2):22-7.

[3] Spear M. Acute or chronic? What's the difference? Plastic Surgical Nursing. 2013; 33(2):98-100.

[4] Vuolo J. Wound care made incredibly easy. Lippincott, Williams and Wilkins; 2009.

[5] Jones ML. A short history of the development of wound care dressings. British Journal of Healthcare Assistants. 2015; 9(10):482-5.

[6] Uzun M. A review of wound management materials. Journal of Textile Engineering & Fashion Technology. 2018; 4(1):00121.

[7] Majno G. The healing hand: Man and wound in the ancient world. Harvard University Press; 1991.

[8] Ovington LG. The evolution of wound management: ancient origins and advances of the past 20 years. Home Healthcare Now. 2002; 20(10):652-6.

[9] George Broughton II, Janis JE, Attinger CE. A brief history of wound care. Plastic and reconstructive surgery. 2006; 117(7S):6S-11S.

[10] Rovee DT. Evolution of wound dressings and their effects on the healing process. Clinical materials. 1991; 8(3-4):183-8.

[11] Shah JB. The history of wound care. The Journal of the American College of Certified Wound Specialists. 2011; 3(3):65-6.

[12] Ahmad W, Aquil Z, Alam SS. Historical background of wound care. Hamdan Medical Journal. 2020; 13(4):189.

[13] Daunton C, Kothari S, Smith L, Steele D. A history of materials and practices for wound management. Wound Practice & Research: Journal of the Australian Wound Management Association. 2012; 20(4).

[14] Forrest RD. Early history of wound treatment. Journal of the Royal Society of Medicine. 1982;7 5(3):198.

[15] Fuchs C, Pham L, Henderson J, Stalnaker KJ, Anderson RR, Tam J. Multi-faceted enhancement of full-thickness skin wound healing by treatment with autologous micro skin tissue columns. Scientific reports. 2021; 11(1):1-3.2

[16] Ehrenfried A. Reverdin and Other Methods of Skin-Grafting: Historical. The Boston Medical and Surgical Journal 1909; 161(26):911-7.

[17] Ang GC. History of skin transplantation. Clinics in Dermatology. 2005; 23(4):320-4.

[18] Hauben DJ, Baruchin A, Mahler A. On the history of the free skin graft. Annals of Plastic Surgery 1982; 9(3):242-5.

[19] Hattery E, Nguyen T, Baker A, Palmieri T. Burn Care in the 1800s. Journal of Burn Care & Research 2015; 36(1):236-9.

[20] McDowell F. Successful attempt of reconstruction of a nose from a completely separated piece of skin from

the leg, by Bünger, Marburg, Germany (Journal der Chirurgie and Augenheilkunde, 4: 569, 1822). Translated from German by Hans May, Plastic and reconstructive surgery 1969; 44(5):486-90.

[21] Fariña-Perez LA. Jaques-Louis Reverdin (1842-1929): The surgeon and the needle. Archivos espanoles de urologia. 2010; 63(4):269-74.

[22] Freshwater MF, Krizek TJ. Skin grafting of burns: A centennial. J Trauma 1971; 11(862):4.

[23] Freshwater MF, Krizek TJ. George David Pollock and the development of skin grafting. Annals of Plastic Surgery. 1978; 1(1):96-102.

[24] Kohlhauser M, Luze H, Nischwitz SP, Kamolz LP. Historical evolution of skin grafting: A Journey through time. Medicina 2021; 57(4):348.

[25] Shimizu R, Kishi K. Skin graft. Plastic Surgery International. 2012; 2012.

[26] Vyas KS, Vasconez HC. Wound healing: Biologics, skin substitutes, bio-membranes and scaffolds. In Healthcare 2014 (Vol. 2, No. 3, pp. 356-400). Multidisciplinary Digital Publishing Institute.

[27] Orgill DP. Excision and skin grafting of thermal burns. New England Journal of Medicine. 2009; 360(9):893-901.

[28] Browne Jr EZ. Complications of skin grafts and pedicle flaps. Hand clinics 1986; 2(2):353-9.

[29] Reddy S. The incidence and risk factors for lower limb skin graft failure. Dermatology Research and Practice 2014.

[30] Kimata Y, Uchiyama K, Ebihara S, Sakuraba M, Iida H, Nakatsuka T, Harii K. Anterolateral thigh flap donor-site complications and morbidity. Plastic and reconstructive surgery. 2000; 106(3):584-9.

[31] Enshaei A, Masoudi N. Survey of Early Complications of Primary Skin Graft and Secondary Skin Graft (Delayed) Surgery after Resection of Burnwaste in Hospitalized Burn Patients. Global journal of health science. 2014; 6(7):98.

[32] Reddy S, El-Haddawi F, Fancourt M, Farrant G, Gilkison W, Henderson N, Kyle S, Mosquera D. The incidence and risk factors for lower limb skin graft failure. Dermatology research and practice. 2014; 2014.

[33] Turissini JD, Elmarsafi T, Evans KK, Kim PJ. Major risk factors contributing to split thickness skin graft failure. Georgetown Medical Review. 2019; 3(1):7755.

[34] Isitt CE, McCloskey KA, Caballo A, Sharma P, Williams A, Leon-Villapalos J, Vizcaychipi MP. An analysis of surgical and anaesthetic factors affecting skin graft viability in patients admitted to a Burns Intensive Care Unit. Scars, Burns & Healing 2016; 2:2059513116642089.

[35] Talbot TR, Schaffner W. Relationship between age and the risk of surgical site infection: A contemporary re-examination of a classic risk factor. J Infec Dis 2005; 191(7): 1032-5.

[36] Schultz G, Mozingo D, Romanelli M, Claxton K. Wound healing and TIME; new concepts and scientific applications. Wound Repair and Regeneration 2005; 13(4): S1-1.

[37] Harries RL, Bosanquet DC, Harding KG. Wound bed preparation: TIME for an update. International Wound Journal. 2016; 13(S3):8-14.

[38] Barrientos S, Stojadinovic O, Golinko MS, Brem H, Tomic-Canic M. Growth factors and cytokines in wound

healing. Wound Repair and Regeneration 2008; 16(5):585-601.

[39] Mast BA, Schultz GS. Interactions of cytokines, growth factors, and proteases in acute and chronic wounds. Wound Repair and Regeneration. 1996; 4(4):411-20.

[40] Wallace HA, Basehore BM, Zito PM. Wound healing phases. In: StatPearls [Internet]. Treasure Island (FL): StatPearls Publishing; 2021.

[41] Brian W. Contribution to the knowledge of the Snakeheads of Iran (Family Channidae). Iran. J. Ichthyol 2016; 3(1):65-72.

[42] Kok LW. Snakeheads – their biology and culture. Recent Advances in Aquaculture. 1982; 180-213.

[43] Das M, Chakraborty SC, Ahmed F, Basak RK. Predatory behaviour of a snakehead fish (Channa striatus Bloch). Bangladesh Journal of Fisheries Research 1998; 2(2):127-37.

[44] Courtenay WR, Williams JD. Snakeheads (Pisces: Channidae): A biological synopsis and risk assessment. United States Geological Survey 2004; United US Department of Interior.

[45] Christy MT, Kirkpatrick W. Indicative 10 Project Extension Material: Striped snakehead (*Channa striata*) 2017; Department of Primary Industries and Regional Development.

[46] Qin J, Fast AW, DeAnda D, Weidenbach RP. Growth and survival of larval snakehead (Channa striatus) fed different diets. Aquaculture. 1997; 148(2-3):105-13.

[47] Qin JG, Fast AW. Food selection and growth of young snakehead Channa striatus. Journal of Applied Ichthyology 1997; 13(1):21-5.

[48] Radzak HA, Akim AM, Sazali SS, Baharum Z, Nata DH, Jalil AA, Sharimala T, Sumasundram AM, Mokhtaruddin N. Total phenolic content, antioxidant, cytotoxicity and hepatoprotective activities of aqueous extract of Channa striatus (Haruan). IOSR Journal of Nursing and Health Science (IOSR-JNHS) 2014; 3(6):52-9.

[49] Jais AM. Pharmacognosy and pharmacology of Haruan (Channa striatus), a medicinal fish with wound healing properties. Boletín Latinoamericano y del Caribe de Plantas Medicinales y Aromáticas. 2007; 6(3):52-60.

[50] Shafri M, Abdul Manan MJ. Therapeutic potential of the Haruan (Channa striatus): from food to medicinal uses. Malaysian Journal of Nutrition. 2012; 18(1):125-36.

[51] Ahmad NI, Wan Mahiyuddin WR, Tengku Mohamad TR, Ling CY, Daud SF, Hussein NC, Abdullah NA, Shaharudin R, Sulaiman LH. Fish consumption pattern among adults of different ethnics in Peninsular Malaysia. Food & Nutrition Research. 2016; 60(1):32697.

[52] Haemamalar K, Zalilah MS, Neng Azhanie A. Nutritional status of orang asli (che wong tribe) adults in Krau Wildlife Reserve, Pahang. Malaysian Journal of Nutrition. 2010; 16(1):555-68.

[53] Aris T, Ahmad NA, Tee GH, editors. National health and morbidity survey 2014: Malaysian Adults Nutrition Survey (MANS). Institute For Public Health; 2014.

[54] Jamaludin SS. Postpartum food restriction of rural Malay women. Asian Journal of Humanities and Social Sciences (AJHSS). 2014; 2(4):32-41.

[55] Poh BK, Wong YP, Karim NA. Postpartum dietary intakes and food taboos among Chinese women attending maternal and child health clinics and maternity hospital, Kuala Lumpur.

Malaysian Journal of Nutrition. 2005; 11(1):1-21.

[56] Jais AM, McCulloch R, Croft K. Fatty acid and amino acid composition in Haruan as a potential role in wound healing. General Pharmacology: The Vascular System. 1994; 25(5):947-50.

[57] Musa AF, Dillion J, Taib ME, Yunos AM, Baie S, Nordin RB. A study on the effect of Haruan fish extract (Channa striatus) on wound healing and quality of life of coronary artery bypass grafting (CABG) patients: A prospective, double-blind, randomized, controlled trial. F1000Research 2018; 7(469):469.

[58] Ab Wahab SZ, Abdul Kadir A, Nik Hussain NH, Omar J, Yunus R, Baie S, Mohd Noor N, Hassan II, Wan Mahmood WH, Abd Razak A, Wan Yusoff WZ. The effect of Channa striatus (Haruan) extract on pain and wound healing of post-lower segment caesarean section women. Evidence-Based Complementary and Alternative Medicine. 2015; 2015:849647.

[59] Marimuthu K, Thilaga M, Kathiresan S, Xavier RH, Mas RH. Effect of different cooking methods on proximate and mineral composition of striped snakehead fish (Channa striatus, Bloch). Journal of food science and technology. 2012; 49(3):373-7.

[60] Engku Hanisah EU, Etty Syarmila IK, Farahniza Z, Norhasidah S, Abdul Salam B, Maaruf AG. Comparative Studies of Antioxidant Activities between Edible Bird Nest, Chicken and Snakehead Fish Soups. Department of Food Science, School of Chemical Sciences and Food Technology, Faculty of Science and Technology, Universiti Kebangsaan Malaysia; 2014.

[61] Laila L, Febriyenti F, Salhimi SM, Baie S. Wound healing effect of Haruan (Channa striatus) spray. International wound journal. 2011; 8(5):484-91.

[62] Abedi S, Far FE, Hussain MK. Effects of Haruan (Channa striatus) Based Cream on Acute. Research Journal of Biological Sciences. 2012; 7(4):181-7.

[63] Febriyenti NA, Baie S. Formulation of aerosol concentrates containing Haruan (Channa striatus) for wound dressing. Malaysian Journal of Pharmaceutical Sciences. 2008; 6(1):43-58.

[64] Febriyenti F, Noor AM, Baie SB. Physical evaluations of Haruan spray for wound dressing and wound healing. International Journal of Drug Delivery 2011; 3(1):115-24.

[65] Hong LW, Theyveeka Selvy A, Rajoo P, Yuan OY, Liong AK, Nair D, Mohamed AF, Zainal Z, Rosli N. Channa Striatus effectiveness in wound-healing: A Scoping Review. IJRAR-International Journal of Research and Analytical Reviews (IJRAR) 2020; 7(1):300-8.

[66] Jerônimo MS, Barros AD, MoritaI VE, Alves EO, Souza NL, Almeida RM, Nóbrega YK, Cavalcanti Neto FF, Amorin R, Borin MD, Bocca AL. Oral or topical administration of L-arginine changes the expression of TGF and iNOS and results in early wounds healing. Acta cirurgica brasileira 2016; 31(9):586-96.

[67] Rahman MA, Molla MH, Sarker MK, Chowdhury SH, Shaikh MM. Snakehead fish (*Channa striata*) and its biochemical properties for therapeutics and health benefits. SF J Biotechnol Biomed Eng 2018; 1(1):1005.

[68] Haniffa MA, Sheela PA, Kavitha K, Jais AM. Salutary value of Haruan, the striped snakehead Channa striatus – a review. Asian Pacific Journal of Tropical Biomedicine. 2014; 4:S8-15.

[69] Chyun JH, Griminger P. Improvement of nitrogen retention by arginine and glycine supplementation

and its relation to collagen synthesis in traumatized mature and aged rats. The Journal of Nutrition. 1984; 114(9):1697-704.

[70] Gam LH, Leow CY, Baie S. Amino acid composition of snakehead fish (Channa striatus) of various sizes obtained at different times of the year. Malaysian Journal of Pharmaceutical Sciences 2005; 3(2):19-30.

[71] Bowman WC, Rand MJ. Textbook of Pharmacology. Blackwell Scientific Publications; 1980.

[72] Gibson RA. Australian fish—An excellent source of both arachidonic acid and ω-3 polyunsaturated fatty acids. Lipids 1983; 18(11):743-52.

[73] Jais AM, Matori MF, Kittakoop P, Sowanborirux K. Fatty acid compositions in mucus and roe of Haruan, Channa striatus, for wound healing. General Pharmacology: The Vascular System. 1998; 30(4):561-3.

[74] Zuraini A, Somchit MN, Solihah MH, Goh YM, Arifah AK, Zakaria MS, Somchit N, Rajion MA, Zakaria ZA, Jais AM. Fatty acid and amino acid composition of three local Malaysian Channa spp. fish. Food Chemistry 2006; 97(4):674-8.

[75] Leaf A, Weber PC. Cardiovascular effects of n-3 fatty acids. New England Journal of Medicine 1988; 318(9):549-57.

[76] Rahnan SA, Huah TS, Nassan O, Daud NM. Fatty acid composition of some Malaysian freshwater fish. Food chemistry 1995; 54(1):45-9.

[77] Ngui WS, Hassan NH, Ramlan N, Zubairi SI. Malaysia snakehead Channa striatus and micropeltes: Physico-chemical properties of fillet fish oil and water-soluble extract. Chemical Engineering Transactions. 2017; 56:61-6.

[78] Heimann W. Fundamentals of Food Chemistry. Prentice Hall Europe 1980.

[79] Lands WE. Fish and Human Health. Academic Press Inc., 1986.

[80] Liu E, Shailaja S, Hoo BS, Mat Jais AM, Lee TL. Thromboelastographic Assessment of the Effect of Snakehead Fish Extracts on Whole Blood Coagulation. InProc. Anaesthesia General Scientific Symposium 2001.

[81] Wang S, Wang Y, Ma J, Ding Y, Zhang S. Phosvitin plays a critical role in the immunity of zebrafish embryos via acting as a pattern recognition receptor and an antimicrobial effector. Journal of Biological Chemistry 2011; 286(25):22653-64.

[82] Subramanian S, Ross NW, MacKinnon SL. Comparison of antimicrobial activity in the epidermal mucus extracts of fish. Comparative Biochemistry and Physiology Part B: Biochemistry and Molecular Biology 2008; 150(1):85-92.

[83] Bhatt P, Kumaresan V, Palanisamy R, Ravichandran G, Mala K, Amin SN, Arshad A, Yusoff FM, Arockiaraj J. A mini review on immune role of chemokines and its receptors in snakehead murrel Channa striatus. Fish & shellfish immunology 2018; 72:670-8.

[84] Das S, Ward LR, Burke C. Prospects of using marine actinobacteria as probiotics in aquaculture. Applied microbiology and biotechnology 2008; 81(3):419-29.

[85] Tiralongo F, Messina G, Lombardo BM, Longhitano L, Li Volti G, Tibullo D. Skin Mucus of Marine Fish as a Source for the Development of Antimicrobial Agents. Frontiers in Marine Science 2020; 7:760.

[86] Dash S, Das SK, Samal J, Thatoi HN. Epidermal mucus, a major determinant in fish health: A review. Iranian Journal of Veterinary Research. 2018; 19(2):72.

[87] Arockiaraj J, Gnanam AJ, Muthukrishnan D, Gudimella R,

Milton J, Singh A, Muthupandian S, Kasi M, Bhassu S. Crustin, a WAP domain containing antimicrobial peptide from freshwater prawn *Macrobrachium rosenbergii*: Immune characterization. Fish & Shellfish Immunology 2013; 34(1):109-18.

[88] Arasu A, Kumaresan V, Sathyamoorthi A, Palanisamy R, Prabha N, Bhatt P, Roy A, Thirumalai MK, Gnanam AJ, Pasupuleti M, Marimuthu K. Fish lily type lectin-1 contains β-prism architecture: Immunological characterization. Molecular Immunology 2013; 56(4):497-506.

[89] Ingram GA. Substances involved in the natural resistance of fish to infection–a review. Journal of Fish Biology 1980; 16(1):23-60.

[90] Ellis AE. Immunity to bacteria in fish. Fish & Shellfish Immunology 1999; 9(4):291-308

[91] Kumari U, Nigam AK, Mitial S, Mitial AK. Antibacterial properties of the skin mucus of the freshwater fishes, *Rita rita* and *Channa punctatus*. European Review for Medical and Pharmacological Sciences 2011; 15(7):781-6.

[92] Reverter M, Tapissier-Bontemps N, Lecchini D, Banaigs B, Sasal P. Biological and ecological roles of external fish mucus: a review. Fishes 2018; 3(4):41.

[93] Austin B, McIntosh D. Natural antibacterial compounds on the surface of rainbow trout, Salmo gairdneri Richardson. Journal of Fish Diseases 1988; 11(3):275-7.

[94] Bragadeeswaran S, Priyadharshini S, Prabhu K, Rani SR. Antimicrobial and haemolytic activity of fish epidermal mucus *Cynoglossus arel* and *Arius caelatus*. Asian Pacific Journal of Tropical Medicine 2011; 4(4):305-9.

[95] Kuppulakshmi C, Prakash M, Gunasekaran G, Manimegalai G, Sarojini S. Antibacterial properties of fish mucus from. European Review for Medical and Pharmacological Sciences. 2008; 12:149-53.

[96] Hellio C, Pons AM, Beaupoil C, Bourgougnon N, Le Gal Y. Antibacterial, antifungal and cytotoxic activities of extracts from fish epidermis and epidermal mucus. International Journal of Antimicrobial Agents 2002; 20(3):214-9.

[97] Bragadeeswaran S, Thangaraj S. Hemolytic and antibacterial studies on skin mucus of eel fish, *Anguilla anguilla* Linnaues, 1758. Asian J Biol Sci 2011; 4(3):272-6.

[98] Rao V, Marimuthu K, Kupusamy T, Rathinam X, Arasu MV, Al-Dhabi NA, Arockiaraj J. Defense properties in the epidermal mucus of different freshwater fish species. Aquaculture, Aquarium, Conservation & Legislation 2015; 8(2):184-94.

[99] Mat Jais AM, Zakaria ZA, Luo A, Song YX. Antifungal activity of Channa striatus (Haruan) crude extracts. International Journal of Tropical Medicine 2008; 3(3):43-8.

[100] Dhanaraj M, Haniffa MA, SV AS, Manikandaraja D. Antibacterial activity of skin and intestinal mucus of five different freshwater fish species viz., Channa striatus, *C. micropeltes*, *C. marulius*, *C. punctatus* and *C. gachua*. Malaysian Journal of Science 2009; 28(3):257-62.

[101] Wei OY, Xavier R, Marimuthu K. Screening of antibacterial activity of mucus extract of snakehead fish, Channa striatus (Bloch). European Review for Medical and Pharmacological Sciences 2010; 14(8):675-81.

[102] Allameh SK, Daud H, Yusoff FM, Saad CR, Ideris A. Isolation,

identification and characterization of Leuconostoc mesenteroides as a new probiotic from intestine of snakehead fish (Channa striatus). African Journal of Biotechnology. 2012; 11(16):3810-6.

[103] Kumar NP, Marimuthu K, Rao RV, Xavier R, Kathiresan S, Suresh CV, Sreeramanan S. Antimicrobial activity of different tissues of snakehead fish Channa striatus (Bloch). Asian Pacific Journal of Tropical Disease. 2012; 2:S302-5.

[104] Zawawi NZ, Shaari R, Nordin ML, Hamdan RH, Peng TL, Zalati CS. Antibacterial and cytotoxic activity assessment of Channa striatus (Haruan) extract. Veterinary World 2020; 13(3):508.

[105] Guo SA, DiPietro LA. Factors affecting wound healing. Journal of Dental Research 2010; 89(3):219-29.

[106] Healy B, Freedman A. Infections. BMJ 2006; 332(7545):838-41.

[107] Yao K, Bae L, Yew WP. Post-operative wound management. Australian Family Physician 2013; 42(12):867-70.

[108] Woo KY. Exploring the effects of pain and stress on wound healing. Advances in Skin & Wound Care 2012; 25(1):38-44.

[109] Pediani R. What has pain relief to do with acute surgical wound healing. World Wide Wounds 2001; 50(2):76.

[110] Muldoon J. Pain, inflammation and wound healing. Nurse Prescribing. 2017; 15(Sup10):14-8.

[111] Brown A. Strategies to reduce or eliminate wound pain. Nursing Times 2014; 110(15):12-5.

[112] Jais AM, Dambisya YM, Lee TL. Antinociceptive activity of Channa striatus (Haruan) extracts in mice. Journal of Ethnopharmacology 1997; 57(2):125-30.

[113] Solihah MH, Israf DA, Zuraini A, Arifah AK, Zakaria MS, Zakaria ZA, Sulaiman MR, Jais AM, Somchit N. Analgesic activity of three Channa spp. fish extracts. Oriental Pharmacy and Experimental Medicine 2006; 6(4):349-54.

[114] Zakaria ZA, Mat Jais AM, Goh YM, Sulaiman MR, Somchit MN. Amino acid and fatty acid composition of an aqueous extract of Channa striatus (Haruan) that exhibits antinociceptive activity. Clinical and Experimental Pharmacology and Physiology 2007; 34(3):198-204.

[115] Dambisya YM, Lee TL, Sathivulu V, Jais AM. Influence of temperature, pH and naloxone on the antinociceptive activity of Channa striatus (Haruan) extracts in mice. Journal of Ethnopharmacology 1999; 66(2):181-6.

[116] Rahnan SA, Huah TS, Nassan O, Daud NM. Fatty acid composition of some Malaysian freshwater fish. Food Chemistry 1995; 54(1):45-9.

[117] Asfar M, Tawali AB, Abdullah N, Mahendradatta M. Extraction of albumin of snakehead fish (Channa striatus) in producing the fish protein concentrate (FPC). International Journal of Scientific & Technology Research 2014; 3(4):85-8.

[118] Asfar M, Tawali AB, Pirman P, Mahendradatta M. Ekstraksi Albumin Ikan Gabus (*Channa striata*) Pada Titik Isoeletriknya. Jurnal Agercolere 2019; 1(1):6-12.

[119] Mustafa A, Widodo MA, Kristianto Y. Albumin and zinc content of snakehead fish (*Channa striata*) extract and its role in health. IEESE International Journal of Science and Technology 2012; 1(2):1.

[120] Borkow G, Melamed E. Copper, An Abandoned Player Returning to the Wound Healing Battle. InTech Open 2021.

[121] Coger V, Million N, Rehbock C, Sures B, Nachev M, Barcikowski S, Wistuba N, Strauß S, Vogt PM. Tissue concentrations of zinc, iron, copper, and magnesium during the phases of full thickness wound healing in a rodent model. Biological Trace Element Research 2019; 191(1):167-76.

[122] Arendsen LP, Thakar R. Basset P, Sultan AH. The impact of copper impregnated wound dressings on surgical site infection following caesarean section: A double-blind randomised controlled study. Eur J Obstet Gynaecol Reprod Biol 2020; 251:83-8.

[123] Lin PH, Sermersheim M, Li H, Lee PH, Steinberg SM, Ma J. Zinc in wound healing modulation. Nutrients 2018; 10(1):16.

[124] Marriage-Arcari R. The role of Zinc in wound healing. Journal of Wound Care Canada 2016; 14(3):18-22.

[125] Rosmawati EA, Tawali AB, MI MS. Chemical Composition, Amino Acid, and Collagen Content of Snakehead (Channa stiata) Fish Skin and Bone. Scientific Research Journal 2018; 6(1):1-4.

[126] Abustam E, Tawali AB, Said MI, Sari DK. Effect of body weight on the chemical composition and collagen content of snakehead fish *Channa striata* skin. Fisheries Science 2018; 84(6):1081-9.

[127] Kwan SH, Baie S, Ismail MN. Profiling of proteins and post translational modifications of Channa striatus dried meat. Current Proteomics 2016; 13(1):9-19.

[128] Kwan SH, Baie S, Mohammed N, Ismail MN. Proteomic profiling of freeze- and spray-dried water extracts of snakehead fish (Channa striatus): In search of biomolecules for wound healing properties. S Asian J Life Sci 2015; 3(1): 22-41.

[129] Hassan SA, Rosnelifaizur R, Maya YM, Samarendra SM, Saringat B, Naing NN, Wan-Arfah N. Effect of oral Channa striatus in laparotomy wound healing of malnourished rats. International Medical Journal 2020; 27(1):67-70.

[130] Baie SH, Sheikh KA. The wound healing properties of Channa striatus-cetrimide cream—tensile strength measurement. Journal of Ethnopharmacology 2000;71(1-2):93-100.

[131] Baie SH, Sheikh KA. The wound healing properties of Channa striatus-cetrimide cream-wound contraction and glycosaminoglycan measurement. Journal of Ethnopharmacology 2000; 73(1-2):15-30.

[132] Rangaraj A, Harding K, Leaper D. Role of collagen in wound management. Wounds 2011; 7(2):54-63.

[133] Chattopadhyay S, Raines RT. Collagen-based biomaterials for wound healing. Biopolymers 2014; 101(8):821-33.

[134] Harsha L, Brundha MP. Role of collagen in wound healing. Drug Invention Today 2020; 13(1).

[135] Woo KY. Exploring the effects of pain and stress on wound healing. Advances In Skin & Wound Care 2012; 25(1):38-44.

[136] Newbern S. Identifying pain and effects on quality of life from chronic wounds secondary to lower-extremity vascular disease: an integrative review. Advances In Skin & Wound Care 2018; 31(3):102-8.

[137] Price P, Krasner DL. Health-related quality of life and chronic wounds:

Evidence and implications for practice. Chronic Wound Care. HMP Communications. 2012: 77-84.

[138] Bakar MR, Kadir AA, Wahab SZ, Karim AH, Hussain NH, Noor NM, Omar J, Baie SB, Mahmood WH, Razak AA, Yunus R. Randomized controlled trial on the effect of Channa striatus extract on measurement of the uterus, pulsatility index, resistive index of uterine artery and superficial skin wound artery in post lower segment caesarean section women. PloS One 2015; 10(7):e0133514.

[139] Braza ME, Fahrenkopf MP. Split-thickness skin grafts. In StatPearls [Internet]; 2020.

[140] Kwan SH, Abdul Aziz NHK, Ismail MN. Bioactive proteins in *Channa striata* promote wound healing through angiogenesis and cell proliferation. Protein & Peptide Letters 2020; 27(1):48-59.

[141] Oosthuizen B, Mole T, Martin R, Myburgh JG. Comparison of standard surgical debridement versus the VERSAJET PlusTM Hydrosurgery system in the treatment of open tibia fractures: prospective open label randomized controlled trail. Int J Burns Trauma 2014; 4(2):53-8.

[142] Rudolph R, Klein L. Healing process in skin grafts. Surg Gynaecol Obstet 1973; 136(4):641-54.

[143] Converse JM, Smahel J, Ballantyne DL, Harper AD. Inosculation of vessels o skin graft and host bed: A fortuitous encounter. Br J Plast Surg 1975; 28(4):274-82.

[144] Lindenblatt N, Calcagni M, Contaldo C, Menger MD, Giovanoli P, Vollmar B. A new model for studying the revascularization of skin grafts in vivo: The role of angiogenesis. Plas Reconstr Surg 2008; 122(6):1669-80.

[145] Aghoghovwia OA, Uhunmwangho EJ, Izah SC. Wond healing potentials of some fin fishes. Int J Res Stud Biosci 2018; 6(5):33-39.

[146] Alhajj M, Bansal P, Goyal A. Physiology, granulation tissues. In StatPearls [Internet]; 2020.

[147] Febriyenti F, Noor AM, Baie S. Formulation of aerosol concentrate containing Haruan (Channa striatus) for wound dressing. Mal J Pharm Sci 2008; 6(1): 43-58.

[148] Baie S, Sheikh KA. The wound healing properties of Channa striatus – cetrimide cream – tensile strength measurement. J Ethnopharm 2000; 71(1):93-100.

[149] Laila L, Febriyenti F, Salhimi M, Baie S. Wound healing effect of Haruan (Channa striatus) spray. Itl World J 2011; 8(5):484-91.

[150] Punzi L, Galozzi P, Luisetto R, Favero M, Ramonda R, Oliviero F, Scanu A. Post-traumatic arthritis: overview on pathogenic mechanisms and role of inflammation. RMD Open 2016; 2(2):e000279.

[151] Muhtadi SA, Sutrisna EM. The potential antidiabetic and anti-inflammatory activity of *Zingiber zerumbet* ethanolic extracts and *Channa striata* powder on albino Wistar mice. Drug Invention Today 2019; 12(1):148-53.

[152] Somchit MN, Solihah MH, Israf DA, Zuraini A, Arifah AK, Jais AM. Effects of three local Malaysian Channa spp. fish on chronic inflammation. Oriental Pharmacy and Experimental Medicine 2004; 4(2):91-4.

[153] Azidah AK, Arifah AK, Roslida AH, Jais AM, Omar J, Sadagatullah AN, Ishak A, Noor NM, Musa AT. A randomized, double-blind study comparing multiple doses of Channa

striatus supplementation for knee osteoarthritis. Oriental Pharmacy and Experimental Medicine 2017; 17(4):345-54.

[154] Shafii N, Omar J, Sirajudeen K, Kadir AA, Baie SH, Wahab SZ, Yunus R, Noor NM, Hussein NH, Razak AA, Mahmood WH. Changes in the inflammatory markers with supplementation of Channa striatus extract in post lower segment caesarean section. International Medical Journal 2017; 24(3):268-71.

[155] Al-Saffar FJ, Ganabadi S, Fakuraz S. Response of Channa striatus extract against monosodium iodoacetate induced osteoarthritis in rats. Journal of Animal and Veterinary Advances 2011; 10(4):460-9.

[156] Ganabadi S. 525 Channa striatus extract supplementation significantly increased protein gene product 9.5-immunoreactive nerve fibres compared to *Zingiber officinale* extract in collagenase induced osteaoarthritis. Osteoarthritis and Cartilage 2009; 17:S281-2.

[157] Kadir AA, Ab Wahab SZ, Zulkifli MM, Noor NM, Baie SB, Haron J. The therapeutic effect of oral Channa striatus extract on primary knee osteoarthritis patients. Agro FOOD Industry Hi Tech 2014; 25(3):44-8.

[158] Kadir AA, Kadir AA, Hamid RA, Mat Jais AM, Omar J, Sadagatullah AN, Badrin S, Win TT, KNS Sirajudeen, Salleh A. Evaluation of Chondroprotective Activity of Channa striatus in Rabbit Osteoarthritis Model. Biomed Research International 2019.

[159] Kadir AA. Snakehead fish (Channa Striatus) in the management of osteoarthritis: Clinical research and possible mechanism of action. Chinese Journal of Traditional Medicine. 2018; 1(1):1-7.

[160] Bakar MN, Abdullah B, Mohamad I, Lazim NM, Yahya NK, Kadir AA. Efficacy of snakehead fish (Channa striatus) extract supplementation in allergic rhinitis patients: A randomized double-blind placebo-controlled trial. International Medical Journal 2019; 26(4):297-300.

[161] Susibalan BD, Abdullah B, Lazim NM, Kadir AA. Efficacy of snakehead fish (Channa striatus) in subjects with allergic rhinitis: a randomized controlled trial. Oriental Pharmacy and Experimental Medicine 2018; 18(3):209-15.

[162] Isa II, Bakar SA, Tohid SF, Mat Jais AM. Channa striatus cream down-regulates tumour necrosis factor (TNF)-alpha gene expression and alleviates chronic-like dermatitis in mouse model. Journal of Ethnopharmacology 2016; 194:469-74.

[163] Meera K, Tarita T, Johar A, Bin Mat Jais AM. Topical Channa striatus 5% cream for inflammatory skin conditions: A phase I randomized double-blind, controlled trial. Iranian Journal of Dermatology 2016; 19(3):67-72

[164] Ali Khan MS, Mat Jais AM, Hussain J, Siddiqua F, Gopala Reddy A, Shivakumar P, Madhuri D. Gastroprotective effect of freeze-dried stripped snakehead fish (*Channa striata* Bloch.) aqueous extract against aspirin induced ulcerogenesis in pylorus ligated rats. International Scholarly Research Notices 2014.

[165] Azemi AK, Abd Rahim MH, Mamat SS, Mat Jais AM, Zakaria ZA. Antiulcer activity of methanol-chloroform extract of Channa striatus fillet. Pakistan Journal of Pharmaceutical Sciences 2018; 31(1):143-151.

[166] Arockiaraj J, Palanisamy R, Arasu A, Sathyamoorthi A, Kumaresan V, Bhatt P, Chaurasia MK,

Pasupuleti M, Gnanam AJ. An anti-apoptotic B-cell lymphoma-2 (BCL-2) from Channa striatus: Sequence analysis and delayed and advanced gene expression in response to fungal, bacterial and poly I: C induction. Molecular immunology 2015; 63(2):586-94.

[167] Buhari I, Roslida A, Hidayat M, Mat Jais AM. Haruan Fish Extract as Potential Agent for Cancer Therapy. J. Cancer Sci. Ther 2015; 7:186-9.

[168] Ghassem M, Arihara K, Babji AS, Said M, Ibrahim S. Purification and identification of ACE inhibitory peptides from Haruan (Channa striatus) myofibrillar protein hydrolysate using HPLC–ESI-TOF MS/MS. Food Chemistry 2011; 129(4):1770-7.

[169] Pujiastuti DY, Ghoyatul Amin MN, Alamsjah MA, Hsu JL. Marine organisms as potential sources of bioactive peptides that inhibit the activity of angiotensin I-converting enzyme: a review. Molecules 2019; 24(14):2541.

[170] Abdul Shukkoor MS, Baharuldin MT, Mat Jais AM, Mohamad Moklas MA, Fakurazi S. Antidepressant-like effect of lipid extract of Channa striatus in chronic unpredictable mild stress model of depression in rats. Evidence-Based Complementary and Alternative Medicine 2016.

[171] Abdul Shukkoor MS, Baharuldin MT, Mat Jais AM, Mohamad Moklas MA, Fakurazi S. Antidepressant-like effect of lipid extract of Channa striatus in chronic unpredictable mild stress model of depression in rats. Evidence-Based Complementary and Alternative Medicine 2016.

[172] Holden J. Top tips for skin graft and donor site management. Wound Essentials 2015; 10(2):7-13.

[173] Hierner R, Degreef H, Vranckx JJ, Garmyn M, Massagé P, van Brussel M. Skin grafting and wound healing—the "dermato-plastic team approach". Clinics in Dermatology 2005; 23(4):343-52.

[174] Beldon P. What you need to know about skin grafts and donor site wounds. Wound Essentials 2007; 2:149-55.

[175] Martyniuk CJ, Denslow ND. Exploring androgen-regulated pathways in teleost fish using transciptomics and poroteomics. Integr Comp Biol 2012; 52: 605-704.

[176] Doherty MK, Brownridge P, Owen MA, Davies SJ, Young IS, Whitfield PD. A proteomics strategy for determining the synthesis and degradation rates of individual proteins in fish. J Proteomics 2012; 75(14): 4471-77.

[177] Gam LH, Leow CY, Baie S. Proteomic analysis of snakehead fish (*Channa striata*) muscle tissue. Malaysian J Biochem Mol Biol 2006; 14(1):25-32.

[178] Serini G & Gabbiani G. Mechanisms of myofibroblast activity and phenotypic modulation. Exp Cell Res 1999; 250(2):273-83.

[179] Burridge K & Chrznowska-Wodnicka M. Focal adhesions, contractility, and signalling. Annu Rev Cell Div Biol 1996; 12(1):463-519.

[180] Kreis TE & Birchmeier W. Stress fibre sarcomeres of fibroblasts are contractile. Cell 1980; 22(2):555-61.

[181] Tomasek JJ, Gabbiani G, Hinz B, Chaponnier C, Brown RA. Myofibroblasts and mechano-regulation of connective tissue remodelling. Nat Rev Mol Cell Biol 2002; 3(5):349-63.

[182] Lees JG, Bach CT, O'Neill GM. Interior decoration: Tropomyosin in actin dynamics and cell migration. Cell Adhes Migr 2011; 5(2):181-86.

[183] Reynolds L, Conti F, Lucas M, Grose R, Robinson S, Stone M, Saundees G, Dickson C, Hynes R, Lacy-Hulbert A. Accelerated re-epithelialization in 3-integrin-deficient mice is associated with enhanced TGF-1 signalling. Nat Med 2005; 11(2):167-174.

[184] Lees JG, Ching YW, Adams D, Bach CT, Samuel MS, Kee AJ, Hardeman EC, Gunning P, Cowin AJ, O'Neill GM. Tropomyosin regulates cell migration during skin wound healing. J Invest Dermatol 2013; 133(5):1330-39.

[185] White MJ, Glenn M, Gomer RH. Trypsin potentiates human fibrocyte differentiation. PloS One 2013; 8(8):e70795.

[186] Gudmundsdóttir A & Pálsdóttir HM. Atlantic cod trypsin: From basic research to practical application. Mar Biotechnol 2005; 7(2):77-88.

[187] Termine JD, Belcourt AB, Conn KM, Kleinman H. Mineral and collagen-binding proteins of foetal calf bone. J Biol Chem 1981; 256(20):10403-08.

[188] Postlethwaite AE, Seyer JM, Kand AH. Chemotactic attraction of human fibroblasts to type I, II, and II collagens and collagen-derived peptides. Proc Natl Acad Sci USA; 1978;75(2):871-5.

[189] Gogia PP. The biology of wound healing. Ostomy Wound Manag 1991; 38(9):12,14-6,18-22.

[190] Helary C, Zaria M, Giraud-Guille MM. Fibroblasts within concentrated collagen hydrogels favour chronic skin wound healing. J Tissue Eng Regener Med 2012; 6(3):225-37.

[191] Benjakul S, Nalinanon S, Shahidi F. Fish collagen: Food Biochemistry and Food processing, 2nd Edition; Wiley and Sons: New York 2012, pp. 365-87.

[192] Hayashi Y, Yamada S, Guchi KY, Koyama Z, Ikeda T. 6 Chitosan and fish collagen as biomaterials for regenerative medicine. Adv Food Nutr Res 2021; 65:107.

[193] Hahn K, DeBiasio R, Taylor DL. Patterns of elevated free calcium and calmodulin activation in living cells. Nature 1992; 359(6397):736-38.

[194] Lansdown AB. Calcium: A potential central regulator in wound healing in the skin. Wound Repair Regen 2002; 10(5):271-85.

[195] Bennet RD, Mauer AS, Pittelkow MR, Strehler EE. Calmodulin-like protein upregulates myosin-10 in human keratinocytes and is regulated during epidermal wound healing in vivo. J Invest Dermatol 2009; 129(3):765-69.

[196] Lasdown A, Sampson B, Rowe A. Sequential changes in trace metal, metallothionein, and calmodulin concentrations in healing skin wounds. J Anat 1999; 195(3):375-86.

[197] Szabolcsi V & Celio MR. De novo expression of parvalbumin in ependymal cells in response to brain injury promotes ependymal remodelling and wound repair. GLIA 2014; 63(4):567-94.

[198] Lubec G, Afjehi-Sadat L, Yang JW, John JPP. Searching for hypothetical proteins: Theory and practice based upon original data and literature. Prog Neurobiol 2005; 77(1):90-127.

Section 2

Skin Grafting

Chapter 4

Types of Skin Grafts

Verónica Olvera-Cortés

Abstract

Skin grafting is a useful technique that has been used for a very long time for achieving closure of wounds when it cannot occure in a natural conventional manner. There are different types of grafts according to their origin, thickness and form. There are 3 main types of graftsthat are used to cover wounds: Split-thickness skin grafts, full-thickness skin grafts and composite grafts. Each of them has specific indication and has a unique technique for harvesting. If the graft is not taken care of properly its survival can be compromised and necrosis of the graft can occur. Even though complications may present, skin grafting is still considered a practical approach to repair many type of wounds.

Keywords: Gratf, Skin, Non melanoma skin cancer, surgery, treatment

1. Introduction

A skin graft is a piece of skin of variable thickness without any vascular connection, separated from the donor site, and afterwards transposed over the recepient site which is to be repaired [1].

This technique was used initially in India about 2.500–3.000 years ago by Tilemaker Caste. It was later rediscovered inthe XIX century and was the most used technique during World War I and II. And in 1823 Buenger was the first to describe a succesful intervention by transfering skin from the buttcheek to the nose [1]. It is a basic technique and an option of reconstruction after a tumor resection, in case of ulcers and burned patients [1].

Skin graft execution is simpler than most skin flaps and can be performed in almost any wound with a vascularized bed. One of the great advantages of skin grafts is that they are very variable in size and shape to allow wound closure of wound defects of different sizes. There are many sites that can be donor sites making it easier for the skin to match.

2. Indications

Wound closure should always follow the principles of the reconstructive ladder, which directs the surgeon to use the least complex method of closure to achieve an ideal cosmetic result [2].

Often a graft may be used when healingof a full thickness wound by second intention, a primary closure, or utilization of a local flap are not feasible options [3].

In some instances, grafts can be used in combination with linear repairs or flaps for skin reconstruction surgery. In addition, skin grafts can be used for shallow defects, or in a patient with multiple morbidities who cannot tolerate a more complex or multi-stage repair [4].

IntechOpen

3. Classification

There are many ways in which skin grafts can be classified, based on their origin, thickness, composition, time in which they are performed, geometry and if it meshed or not (**Table 1**).

According to their origin, skin grafts can be divided in 3: Autografts, allografts and xenografts.

Autografts are taken from the patient's own skin, and they are the most common used skin grafts.

Allografts come from another person's skin. And xenograftsare derived from another species, other than human skin, for example porcine grafts. Both allografts and xenografts are used in chronic wounds or burn wounds. Their utility comes from their ability to stimulate wound healing, provide protection and achieve debridement [3].

In terms of thickness, they are distinguished as: Split-thickness skin grafts and full-thickness skin grafts [1] and composite grafts.

Split-thickness skin grafts are composed by epidermis and a variable thickness of dermis. They can be subdivided in 3 [1]:

- Thin: 0.15–0.25 mm
- Intermediate: 0.3–0.4 mm
- Thick: 0.5–0.6 mm

Full-thickness skin grafts are composed of epidermis and dermis with skin appendages [1].

The amount of dermis in the skin graft determines many properties of the graft, such as resistance to pressure and shear forces, shrinkage, sensitibity and esthetic results. In other words, the thicker the graft the better mechanical, functional and aesthethic properties, but also this means that the neo and revascularization of the graft will be more difficult.

If the graft includes other tissue besides skin it is a composite graft. Composite grafts are made by two different tisular structures, skin and cartilage most of the cases [1].

According to the moment in time in which the graft is realized [1]:

Character	**Types**
Origin	1. Autograft 2. Allograft 3. Xenograft
Thickness	1. Split thickness 2. Full thickness 3. Composite
Time	1. Immediate 2. Differed
Expansion	1. Sheet graft 2. Meshed graft

Table 1.
Classification of skin grafts.

Immediate: Realized just after the resection of the tumor. To repair the loss of substance.

Differed: The graft is performed in a second intervention, in order to have the confirmation of clean margins. This approach is justified for agressive tumors and tumor relapse, to obtain granulation tissue when the surgery is extense in depth and/or width, and exceptionally when hemostasis of the reciepent site cannot be achieved [1].

Another way to classify skin grafts is based if a technique is used to expand the graft itself. If the skin graft is directly applied onto the defect without further treatment this is called an unmeshed or sheet graft [5].

A mesh graft is when multiple slits are made on the graft. Usually this is made with a mechanical mesher and it is common to apply this on split-thickness skin grafts. Meek graft is a skin graft that is cut in stripes, equal in lenght and width. It used a cork plate and a machine with rotating blades. Punch grafts are obtained using a punch, which allows to obtain multiple full-thinkcness skin grafts, it is a useful technique to cover large wound areas.

4. Physiology

The survival of skin grafts is a complex process that involves different phases. In order to undestand them it is necessary to remember how the skin is irrigated.

Skin consists of 2 basic layers, the epidermis and dermis. The dermis is divided into a papillary and reticular layer. Within the dermis resides the skin's neurovascular supply. The subcutaneous tissue beneath the skin contains the superficial fascia and subcutaneous fat [6].

The skin vasculature consists of a deep dermal/subcutaneous plexus and a superficial plexus [6]. Both plexi are connected via communicating vessels. The superficial plexus can be found in the reticular dermis, near its junction with the papillary dermis. The deep plexus, located in the subcutaneous tissue, consists of an extensive venous plexus, capable of holding large quantities of blood and an accompanying artery. The deep plexus supplies vessels to the pilosebaceous units and the superficial plexus. Arteriovenous anastomoses also exist in the region [6, 7]. The superficial plexus originates vascular loops within the papillary dermis. Nutrients diffuse into the epidermis because no vessels cross the dermal-epidermal junction. Venous and lymphatic systems exist in a similar arrangement [6].

Unlike flaps, grafts depend on the ingrowth of capillaries from the recipient site for their ultimate survival [8].

For the first 24–48 hours, the graft initially derives oxygen and nutrients from the underlying bed by diffusion (plasmatic diffusion or imbibition). The graft can increase in weight by up to 40%. During imbibition, the graft and the wound bed are held together via a layer of fibrin. The fibrin is eventually replaced by granulation tissue [2, 3, 8].

The second phase, inosculation, is defined by an anastomosis of the preexistent vessels of the graft and the wound base. This phase occurs during the second and third postoperative days [3].

For graft-take tooccur, the recipient site must be capableof producing capillary buds. Since capillaryoutgrowth is needed both to producegranulation tissue and to nourish askin graft, areas that granulate well (muscle and deep fascia), acceptgrafts readily. Other surfaces, such astendon denuded of its fascia covering, exposed bone, or cartilage, are incapableof producing granulation tissue and, therefore, are unable to nourish a skingraft [9].

Also the skingraft must remain in close approximationto the recipient bed during thephase of capillary ingrowth. The presenceof air, serum, or fluid between thegraft and recipient bed creates a barrierthrough which the capillaries cannotgrow fast enough to prevent necrosis ofthe graft [9].

Revascularization involves the growth, proliferation, and connection of vessels from the recipient base and sidewalls. The rate of revascularization is dependent on the thickness of the graft and the vascularity of the recipient bed. As a general rule, the thinner theskin graft, the faster it establishes a blood supply [9].

Within 4 to 7 days, full circulation has been restored to the graft. Restoration of lymphatic circulation also occurs within 7 days. Reinnervation of the graft begins approximately 2 to 4 weeks after grafting; however, full sensation may require several months or even years to return to normal [8].

5. Technique

5.1 Split-thickness skin grafts (STSG)

STSG are indicated for large defects (>5 cm), slow- or nonhealing chronic wounds, or as a temporary cover when monitoring a wound bed for potential cancer recurrence [3, 10].

This type of skin graft is useful when the definitive reconstruction of a wound is delayed, either for surveillance of an aggressive cancer or when granulation tissue is needed on the bed of the recepient site.

Donor site selection is based on the size of the graft needed to cover the wound, the patient's ability to care for the donor site and how the donor site wound would affect the patient's daily activities (walk, sit, sleep). Taking all this in consideration the medial and lateral thighs are most used for donor site. Also it is practical to consider donor sites that can be hiddenunder clothing, such as the medial or lateral upper arm, abdomen, back andbuttocks. Donorsites that offer large flat surfaces also facilitate theharvesting of STSGs [11].

Once the donor area has been selected, it should be shaved of all hair to aid in the harvesting and handling of the skin graft [8].

The donor site should be prepared and draped in the normal sterile fashion and local anesthesia may be infiltrated [4]. If the graft requirement is significant, saline may be infiltrated instead of local anesthesia to make the graft harvesting easier.

STSG may be harvested using a dermatome or the freehand technique, depending on the size of graft needed and location of the recipient site [3].

There are many electric dermatomes available (e.g. Davol, Padgett, Zimmer), all of them with adjustable graft width and thickness.

After marking the dimensions of the graft (mark the skin graft 15–20% larger than needed and thus allow for shrinkage), the skin is lubricated with sterile ointment. The assistant surgeon should keep the skin flat and stretched by countertension [12].

The dermatome is held at a 30° to 45° angle, and advanced, from proximal to distal, while traction is maintained on the skin. Toothless forceps are used to prevent the graft from getting snared, and the dermatome is lifted away while still engaged [10–12].

After the STSG is obtained it is transferred to a sterile-saline soaked gauze to keep it moist. Attention must be paid in order not to confuse the dermal and epidermal surface when handling the skin graft. A useful tip is to remember that the dermal surface glistens more than the epidermal side and also the edges of the graft will curve to the dermal surface.

Meshing the STSG allows the graft to cover a wound that is larger in dimensions than the unmeshed STSG. Meshing increases the coverage area by 25–35% and also increases the flexibility of the graft so it can be used over mobile surfaces such as joints [4].

It also provides fenestrations in the skin graft that allow the egress of fluid from the wound bed, which minimizes the chance of seroma or hematoma formation and subsequent graft failure. Mechanical meshing of grafts is recommended when they are being used to cover defects >8 cm in diameter or when extensive serosanguineous drainage is anticipated [4].

Meshing can be accomplished in a variety of ways, but the most common and efficient method is to use a hand-powered mechanical mesher to produce multiple uniform slits in a skin graft, approximately 0.05 inches apart. The skin to be meshed is placed on a carrier with the dermis side up and spread over the carrier. The graft is then passed through the mesher. It is is then covered with moist saline gauze. Split thickness grafts can be meshed to obtain expansion from 1:1 upto 1:4. In case of paucity of donor site and large recipient area the graft can be meshed to achieve expansion of 1:9. The survival of such widely meshed graft can be improved by covering it with 1: 3 meshed allograft. This methodis called sandwich grafting. Xenograft can also be used for this purpose. The disadvantages of meshing include suboptimal cosmesis and delay in ultimate closure of the grafted site [2, 8].

The donor site should be temporarily covered with gauze soaked in 1% lidocaine with epinephrine while attention is quickly turned back to the graft. The epinephrine in the solution promotes hemostasis in this acute, abrasion-like donor site [4].

The recipient site must be prepared before the placement of the STSG. Since there must be close contact between the skin graft and wound bed, a good hemostasis should be done in order to prevent hematoma formation. If the wound bed has granulated tissue all the fibrinous debris have to be removed.

When the STSG is placed over the recipient site sometimes it needs to be cut to fit the size of the wound. After the graft is trimmed it has to be attached to initiate contact between the graft and the wound bed. In order to achieve this a tie-over dressing is used. First apply an antibiotic impregnated gauze on the graft, after a foam dressing or sponge is putover the gauze, put single sutures around the defect and leave long tails of the sutures, this long tails will be tied over the dressing or sponge.

Attention is subsequently turned to the donor site, which is best treated as a superficial abrasion. Further hemostasis is usually not necessary. A moist occlusive dressing is applied, making use of antibiotic ointment or petrolatum and a nonadherent dressing such aspolymer film [4].

The donor site presents important drainage during the first 48 hrs, this is a normal process and it is important to inform the patient. In order to avoid fluid colection the dressing can be punctured at the site to allow drainage or the dressing can be changed more frequently.

In the postoperative period the most important part is to minimize all physical activity. Since any abrupt or strong movement may affect the graft, shearing forces can be created and the graft itself may be damaged or bleeding from the wound bed can occur. Separation of the graft from the recipient site compromises its vascularization and eventually its survival. This is why the patient is adviced to elevate the intervened area and restrict all physical efforts.

The manipulation of the dressings should be kept at minimum in order to avoid contamination or involuntary movement that may disrupt the process of revascularization of the graft, which takes about 3 to 5 days.

After wound healing is achieved it is important to advice the patient to avoid sunshine and to use sun-blocking agents to prevent hyperpigmentation, use a greasy ointment to reduce dryness and itching [12].

The advantages of using this type of skin graft are: Very easy and fast harvesting, provides good color match in most cases, they may be obtained from any area of the body, provides skin for large defects [12].

The disadvantages of this type of grafts are: Graft contraction and hyperpigmentation (Split thickness grafts will contract 10–20% immediately after harvest and up to 20–50% over time), fixation may be inadequate, leading to shearing and wound dehiscence, cannot be used on exposed tendon, nerves, cartilage, or bone, development of hematoma or seroma may lead to poor vascularization of the graft, in case of wound infection, skin graft may turn necrotic within 24 h [2, 12].

5.2 Full-thickness skin grafts (FTSG)

FTSG are very useful in dermatologic surgery, especially after the removalof a skin cancer, areas that are conducive to FTSG include nasal ala and tip, helix, medial canthus, lower eyelid, digits, and extremities. FTSG should be limited to less than 5 cm [3].

In order to maximize cosmesis, various factors must be taken into account when choosing a site to harvest, including photodamage, color, existing adnexal structures (hair), and the appearance of the donor site scar. Donor skin should be devoid of malignant lesions or any changes that might later be confused for recurrence of malignancy. Commonly used sites for FTSG are: pre- and postauricular regions, creases of the upper eyelids, nasolabial folds, supraclavicular region, lateral neck, antecubital fossa, and groin [3, 8].

Once the appropriate donor site has been chosen, anesthetized, cleansed, and prepared for harvest, a template of the defect is made by using gauze, cardboard labels, or foil from suture packaging. The template is then transposed to the donorsite.

The skin graft will contract at the recepient site, for this reason it is important to make the template 10–20% bigger in order to avoid distortion of the anatomy of the area that was intervened. When eyelids defects are closed using a skin graft the template needs to be oversized more so that ectoprion will not develop.

Full thickness grafts should be harvested at the level just deep to the dermis, not down to fascia, as the graft will need to be thinned [2]. Once the graft is obtained, all the subcutaneous tissue must be removed using curved iris scissors. Remove the adherent fat by putting the graft under tension. Roll the graft overyour forefinger and pull it down with your middle finger and thumb [12]. The goal is to expose the dermis. Since any remaining fat will obstruct the imbibition phase.

Remoistening the graft periodically with sterile saline or local anesthetic during the defatting procedure is recommended to prevent desiccation [11].

Before placing a skin graft, the recipient site must be clean and not actively bleeding [8].

After placing the graft in the recepient site it needs to be fixated with sutures. Optimal suturing technique is with the needle entering the graft first, 2–3 mm from the edge, and then exiting in the adjacent recipient site skin and subsequently tied with 3–4 throws of a square knot. Distance between sutures is usually 3–4 mm [4] (**Figures 1** and **2**).

It is important to place sutures sufficiently deep such that both the papillary and reticular dermis of the graft and recipient site are directly aligned with each other. Suturing that is too superficial apposes only the papillary dermis, leaving a dead space in the deeper reticular dermis which tends to retract more than the superficial papillary dermis. This increases the risk of both hematoma formation and a depressed, more visible scar. Excessively superficial suturing has also been implicated as a potential etiology of graft pin-cushioning [4].

Bolsters are used to stabilize and protect the graft and to provide a uniform pressure dressing to the grafted area. Bolster materials include saline-soaked dental rolls, saline-soaked gauze, and mineral oil–soaked cotton balls. The bolsters should have a nonstick surface and should be fitted to the size of the graft. They are secured with simple interrupted sutures using 4–0 silk are placed in pairs directly across from one another 2–3 mm from the graft margins. Bolsters are left in place for 5 to 7 days [3, 10].

The donor site is repaired later after the graft has been placed as it is important to allow nutrient diffusion to the graft to begin [3].

During the postoperative period the use of antibiotic oinment is recommended for the recipient and donor site in order to avoid infection. Also the dressing in the recipient site has to be checked every day for one week and every 2 to 3 days at the donor site. Both areas have to be cleaned with saline solution. The sutures can be removed after 7–8 days.

Development of pink color during 3 to 7 days signals neovascularization and successful graft take. Over the ensuing 1 to 2 months, pink color diminishes, but the graft may remain lighter than surroundingskin (**Figures 3** and **4**) [10].

The advantages of this technique are: easy and rapid harvesting, provides excellent color match and adequate thickness of the skin, a small scar remains after skin harvesting and primary closure of the donor site [12].

The disadvantages of this type of grafts are: limited size of skin for harvesting, donor site will require STSG when primary closure is not possible [12].

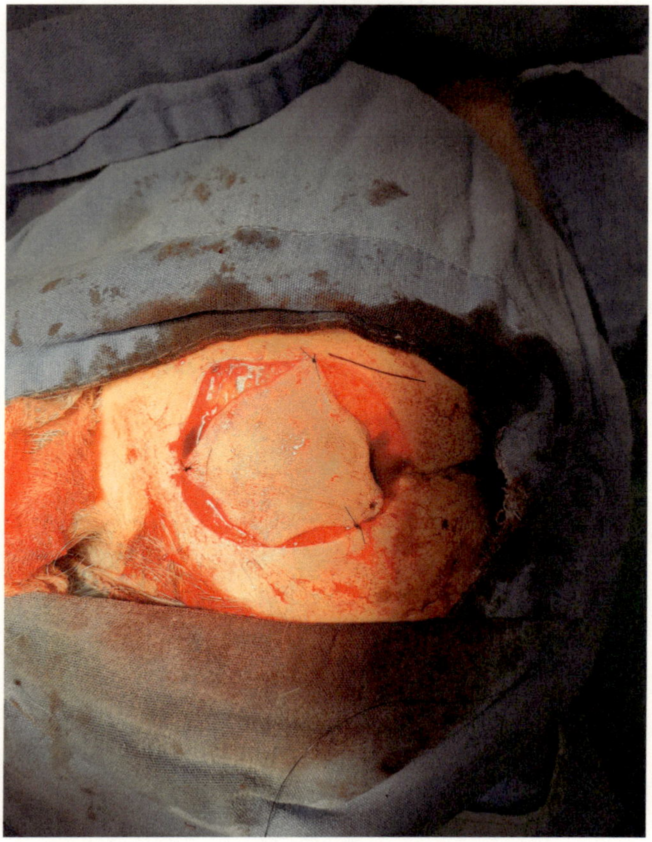

Figure 1.
Initial attachment of the Full-skin graft.

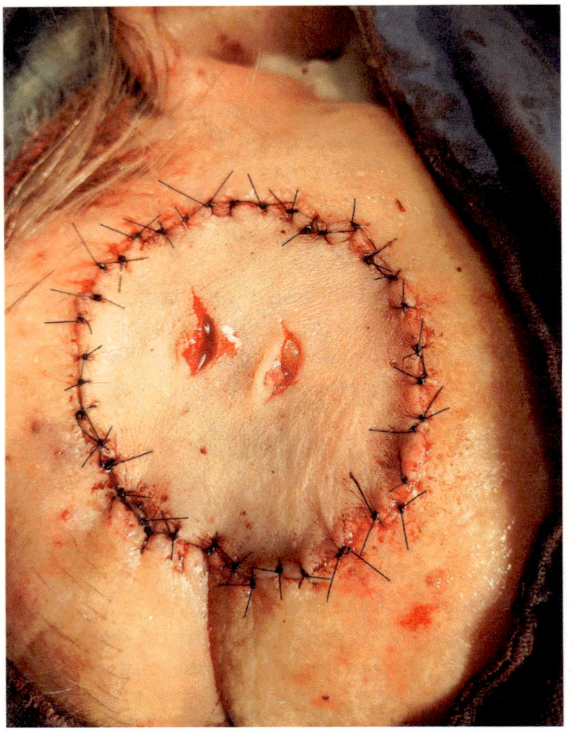

Figure 2.
Complete placement of sutures attaching the FSG.

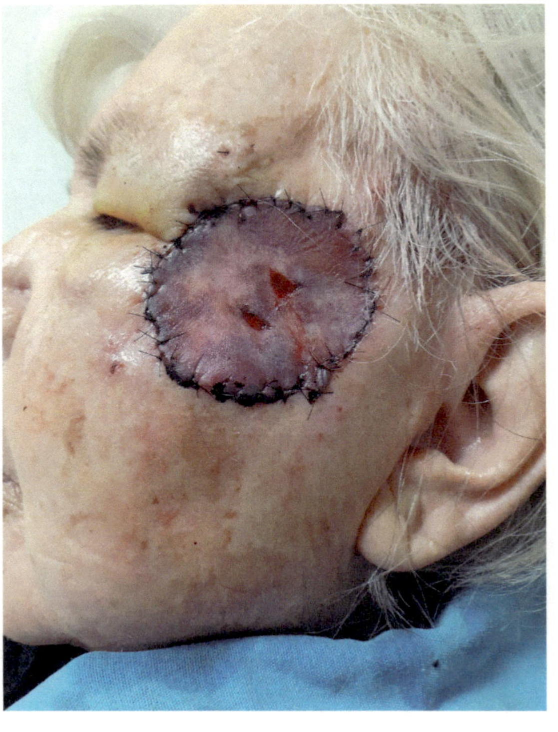

Figure 3.
Full-skin graft appearance after removing the bolster (48 hrs),

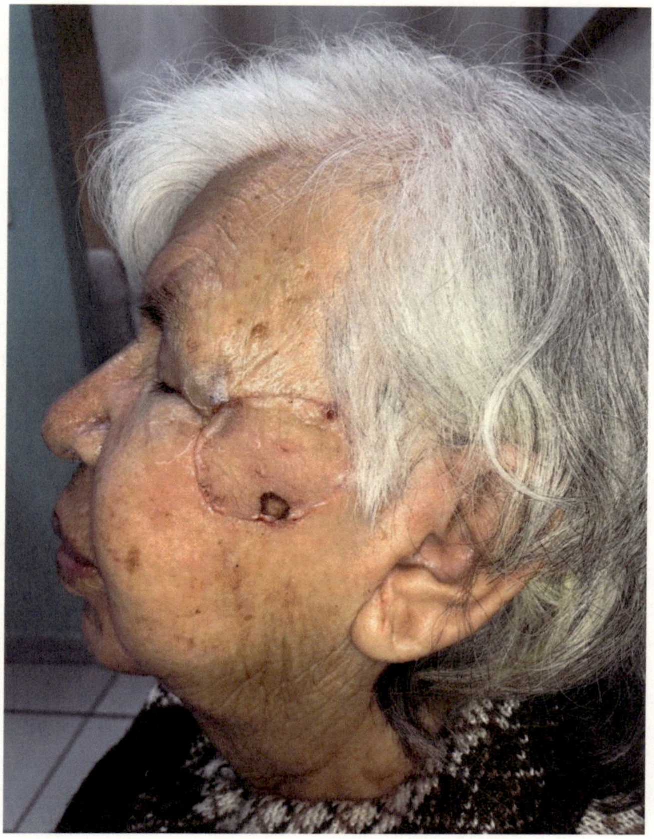

Figure 4.
Full-skin graft appearance at one month after the surgery.

5.3 Composite grafts

This type of graft consists of two different type of tissues. Mostly cartilage with or without subcutaneous tissue and the overlying skin. Because they offer support and structure composite grafts are used to repair full-thickness defects of the nasal ala and helical rim. The size of the defect for this type of graft is 1 cm or less.

They can also beused to fill partial-thickness defects that extend toodeeply for a full-thickness skin graft to heal withoutleaving a concavity or contraction of the free margin [13].

The metabolic needs of composite grafts differ from the needs of skin grafts, the former have greater demands and needs rapid revascularization in order to survive. The blood flow formed by the anastomoses between the wound bed and composite graft can extend only to a small portion beyond the margin of the graft. Portions of the graft that are beyond 1 cm from the vessel anastomoses is at risk of not receiving appropiate blood flow and is at risk of necrosis.

Its survival depends on passivediffusion of oxygen and nutrients through the-perichondrium from adjacent vascularized tissue. The vascularity of the recipient bed is also aconsideration. The nasal ala is generally well suppliedwith blood vessels and can usually support composite grafts [13].

Because the cartilage in these grafts carries with itthe skin that will cover the cutaneous portion of thedefect, the donor site should be chosen so that thetexture, color, and nature of appendages match as best aspossible the features of the recipient site [13].

The ear exhibits a wide range of thicknesses, curvatures, and appendage-type structures [13]. Composite auricular graftsharvested from the helical crus are particularlyuseful, because they provide thin skin that istightly adherent to the underlying cartilage. Thegraft affords structural support and resemblesfine nasal skin being reconstructed [10].

First, the recipient site is measured andthe donor site marked such that the composite graftwill be approximately 5–10% larger than thedefect. This oversizing will compensatefor the natural shrinkage of the graft that occurs during healing [13].

Once the donor site has been closed, the graft isprepared. Using a pair of curved iris scissors, the skinis trimmed from the wings to expose the underlyingcartilage. The remaining cartilaginous pegs shouldframe the lateral aspects of the graft [13]. A hemostat or scissors maybe used to undermine pockets on each side of the defect. These pockets should run parallel to the alar or helicalrim and should only be deep enough to accommodatethe cartilaginous pegs of the composite graft. And the cartilaginouspegs are gently inserted into these pocketsso that the graft interlocks with its recipient bed [13].

The graft is securedin place with a single layer of suture throughskin and perichondrium, minimizing sutures passing through cartilage. Limiting sutures andgraft trauma facilitates robust vessel ingrowth [10].

Antibiotic-impregnated gauze should be placed inthe patient's nostril to stabilize the alar rim. Apressure dressing or bolster should be used to stabilize the graft [13].

In the postoperative perdiod, the intranasal gauze needs to stay for 24-48 hrs and then removed so that the wound can be cleaned. Any activity that may elevate the patient's blood pressure has to be avoided. The sutures can be removed after 7 days.

Composite grafts change their color during the following days after the procedure. At first the graft will be pallid because of tha lack of blood flow. After 6 hrs it changes color to lightly pink, representing the begining of the vessel anastomoses. The next 24–48 hrs the graft becomes blue because of venous congestion that follows, and will remain like this for a week, until venous drainage begins. Later it will become pink and this indicates adequate blood flow and graft survival. The pink color will increase in the next days reaching a red color as the healing process continues. After 2 to 6 months later the red color will disappear. The final tone can be achieved after 1 or 2 years.

6. Complications

All types of grafts can present complications that may compromise it's survival.

Complete or partial graft failure is the primary complicationseen with FTSGs. Causes for failure includehematoma, graft-bed contact disruption, infection, smoking, and excessive electrocoagulation of the wound base [8].

If the skin graft develops necrosis it should not be debrided, the necrotic tissue serves as a natural dressing that allows new skin formation under it. There can be some contour alterations made by the healing process, specially on the nose (elevation), that can improve by themselves in a period of 6 months, if after that period the alterations remain dermabrasion or intralesional steroids can be used.

The acute complications of STSG are the same of those presented by FTSG (hematoma, seroma, graft movement). Long term complications of STSG are related to skin graft contraction that may distort free margins, impair function, develop graft fragility or alter the final aesthethic result.

If infection of the graft is suspected or developed a skin culture needs to be performed and proper antibiotics should be given.

In composite grafts short-term potential complications, includebleeding, infection, and necrosis of the graft. This last complication presents initially as a yellowish whiteness that remains and then is followed by the aparition of a black eschar.

Should the graft become necrotic, the escharshould not be debrided. The necrosis may only besuperficial, with the underlying dermis and cartilage still viable [13].

Long term complications of composite grafts are consequence of an inappropiate anchorage of the graft to the recipient site, trauma or extreme contractural forces, all of which can cause displacement or deformation of the graft.

7. Conclusions

Since their initial use almost 3.000 years ago skin grafts have been a very useful option for wound repair. Whether it is due to an ulcer, burn or surgery, wound closure can be accomplished via skin grafts in any of their modalities. Skin grafts offer a very useful alternative for reconstruction that can be applied to almost any site of the body. It is imperative to select an adequate donor site to offer the best match possible. The process and technique of each type of graft is easy to perfom. And with the correct sterile and surgical technique the possibilty of complications is minimized. This type of wound management should not be considered as a last resort, since their advantages outweigh the disadvantages.

Author details

Verónica Olvera-Cortés
Instituto Mexicano del Seguro Social, Ciudad de México, Mexico

*Address all correspondence to: dra.veronica.olvera@gmail.com

References

[1] Blatière V. Injertos cutáneos: injertos de piel de grosor variable y total. EMC Dermatología. 2021;55(1):1-17.

[2] Jensen AR, Klein MB, Ver Halen JP, Wright AS, Horvath KD. Skin Flaps and Grafts: A Primer for the National Technical Skills Curriculum Advanced Tissue-Handling Module. J Surg Educ. 2008;65(3):191-199.

[3] Leal-Khouri SM and Grummer SE. Skin Grafting. In: Nouri K. Mohs Micrographic Surgery. 1st ed. Springer-Verlag London. 2012. p. 433-442.

[4] Acosta AE, Aasi SZ, MacNeal RJ, Messingham MJ, Arpey CJ. Skin Grafting. In: Robinson JK, Hanke CW, Siegel DM, Fratila A. Surgery of the Skin: Procedural Dermatology. 3rd ed. Saunders Publishing. 2015. p.306-323.

[5] Hierner R, Degreef H, Vranckx JJ, Garmyn M, Massagé P, Van Brussel M. Skin grafting and wound healing—the "dermato-plastic team approach". Clin Dermatol. 2005;23:343-352.

[6] Losquadro WD. Anatomy of the Skin and the Pathogenesis of Nonmelanoma Skin Cancer. Facial Plast Surg Clin N Am. 2017;25:283-289.

[7] Ablove RH, Howell RM. The Physiology And Technique Of Skin Grafting. Hand Clin. 1997;13(2):163-173.

[8] Adams DC, Ramsey ML. Grafts in Dermatologic Surgery: Review and Update on Full- and Split-Thickness Skin Grafts, Free Cartilage Grafts, and Composite Grafts. Dermatol Surg. 2005;31:1055-1067.

[9] Lyons RJ. Promoting healing of skin flaps and grafts. AORN Journal. 1982:35(6):1174-1176.

[10] Brenner MJ, Moyer JS. Skin and Composite Grafting Techniques in Facial Reconstruction for Skin Cancer. Facial Plast Surg Clin N Am. 2017;25: 347-363.

[11] Zhang AY, Meine JG. Flaps and Grafts Reconstruction. Dermatol Clin. 2011;29:217-230.

[12] Erovic BM, Lercher P. Skin Graft Harvesting. In: Erovic BM, Lercher P. Manual of Head and Neck Reconstruction Using Regional and Free Flaps. 1st ed. Springer-Verlag Wien. 2015. p. 53-60.

[13] Adams C, Ratner D. Composite and free cartilage grafting. Dermatol Clin. 2005;23:129-140.

Chapter 5

Skin Graft Fixation and Methods

Sundaram Ravanasamudram Rajaram and Gauthami Sundar

Abstract

Skin graft fixation constitutes the most important element for the success of the reconstruction. The stability of the skin graft over the wound is a determinant factor for its survival. Many techniques have been described in the literature for fixing the skin graft. The most frequent of the techniques is the tie over technique. Staples, fibrin glue are other advancements in the arena of skin graft fixation. The skin graft is covered by a dressing material which keeps it undisturbed and protects the graft from infection. The quest for an ideal dressing material has led to many innovative materials and methods to apply them.

Keywords: history of graft fixation, skin graft fixation, tie over dressing, staples, fibrin glue

1. Introduction

Skin grafting is one of the most commonly done surgical procedures as a part of reconstructive process. The skin grafts are routinely being used in a variety of situations including traumatic wound reconstruction, oncologic reconstruction, cosmetic problems like scar contraction. Skin graft fixation forms a crucial step in the success of the skin grafting. Various techniques of skin graft fixation have been practiced and they have their own advantages and disadvantages.

However, the basic principles of the skin graft fixation remains constant and when satisfied leads to the success of the procedure. Varying situations demand varying type of the skin graft fixation techniques.

The conventional skin graft fixation technique involves pressure application over the skin graft using a bolus and tie over sutures. The skin graft edges are fixed to the recipient bed meticulously using sutures that would be removed later. Over the years, further advancements in graft fixation techniques have been witnessed like the use of staples replacing the sutures, glue for skin graft adhesion and Negative wound therapy. This chapter elaborates the various skin graft fixation techniques and the dressing materials which aid in skin graft healing.

2. History of skin graft fixation techniques

The history of free skin grafting dates back to as early as 600 BC in ancient India where the defects of the ears, nose and lips were treated using free gluteal grafts and skin grafts [1].

Tile maker caste have been known for practicing free skin grafts, harvested from the gluteal region which was prepared by beating with wooden slippers until significant swelling had taken place they also used a secret cement for adhesion of the skin grafts which was called the "ancient Indian method" [2].

The suturing of the skin edges had been carried out by using giant ants, according to Sushrutha Samhitha. The ants were gently allowed to bite across the skin edges to be approximated. As soon as the ant bites well, the body is cut off leaving the head of the ants in place. There are evidences of using thorns to approximate the skin edges too. Similar technique for skin approximation using the ants had been in practice in ancient Egypt also.

It was the 'cisterian monks' in Worcesterschire who made a mark in the history for having used needles and sutures to approximate the wound edges. Evidently after this time scale, the modern day suturing started and securing the skin grafts by sutures come into practice [3].

Bergel in 1909 discussed about the hemostatic nature of fibrin. In 1985, Rose, Dresdale et al. [4] described the combination of fresh frozen plasma and bovine thrombin to form fibrin glue. During the 1990s, the fibrin sealant was widely put into use and became FDA approved. The fibrin also showed adhesive properties that were utilized in cases of fistula closure and seroma prevention. Later it was used as a skin graft fixation agent sometimes replacing sutures and staples [5].

Present day scenario sees the use of sutures, staples and fibrin glues for fixation of the skin grafts.

3. Fixation of skin grafts

The recipient bed interface has a thin fibrin bed that holds the skin graft on to it. The fibrin acts as a barrier against infections that can cause graft failure [6]. Bleeding, shearing force, wound infection can all lead to graft loss, thus necessitating proper anchoring and protective dressing.

The skin graft goes through 2 distinct phases of adherence.

Phase 1: it lasts till 72 hours. The adherence is maintained by fibrin layer.

Phase 2: it commences after 72 hours because of the fibrous ingrowth and vascular anastomoses [7].

3.1 Securing the skin grafts

The skin graft edges are trimmed and the recipient wound edges are undermined to accommodate the skin graft (**Figure 1a–e**). The edges of the skin graft are approximated and secured to the edges of the recipient wound with sutures or staples (**Figure 2a** and **b**). The staples have the added advantage of consuming less time in securing the skin graft edges. There are several operators who wish to place absorbable sutures thereby negating the burden of suture removal after healing [8].

3.2 Dressing over the skin graft

Appropriate dressing is placed over the skin graft for better adaptation and graft healing. This also avoids the seroma formation and hematoma formation that can subsequently lead to infection and graft failure.

3.2.1 Tie over dressing/bolster dressing

The tie over dressing is one of the earliest and effective methods for graft fixation (**Figure 3a** and **b**). Once the graft is transferred to the recipient bed and secured with sutures, a bolster is placed on the skin graft and secured with silk sutures running over the bolster and offering some pressure that prevents dislodgement.
The bolster generally would be a piled up gauze pieces.

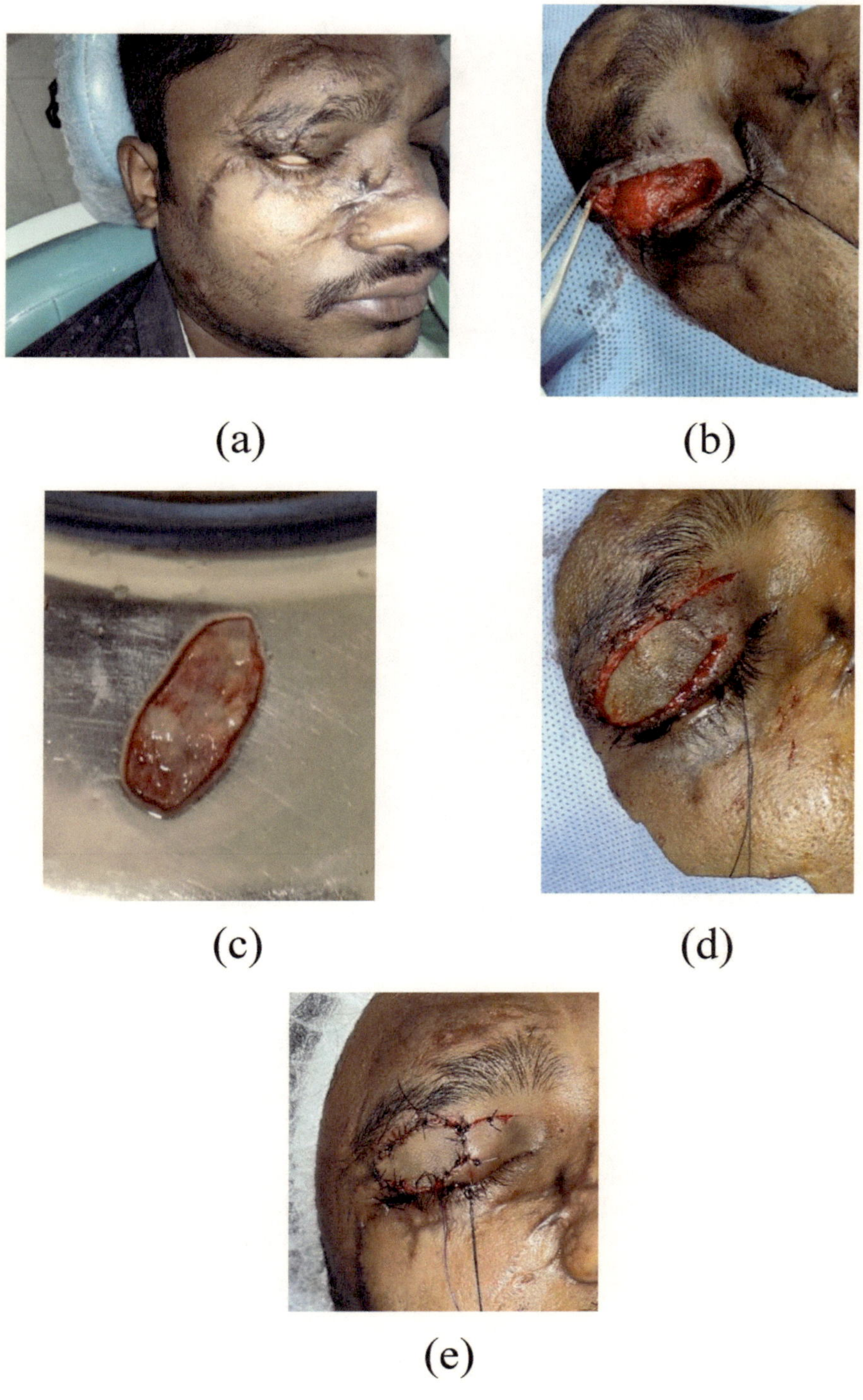

Figure 1.
(a) A case of facial scar. (b) Undermining of wound edges. (c) Skin graft edges trimmed. (d) Skin graft adapted. (e) Skin graft secured with sutures.

Although supported only by some observational studies, the tie over dressing remains simple and effective means for skin graft fixation.

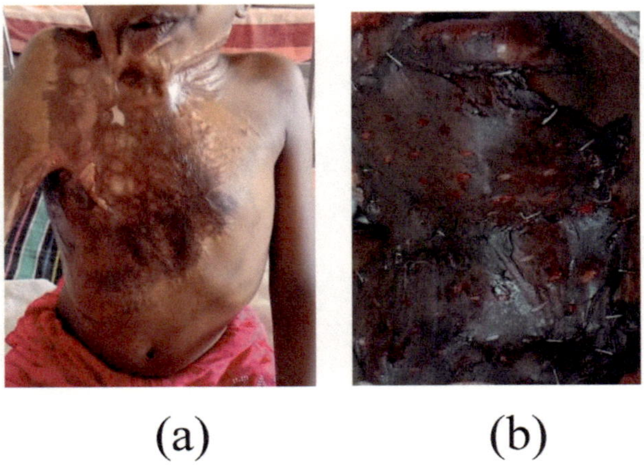

Figure 2.
(a) A case of burns scar. (b) Skin graft secured with staples.

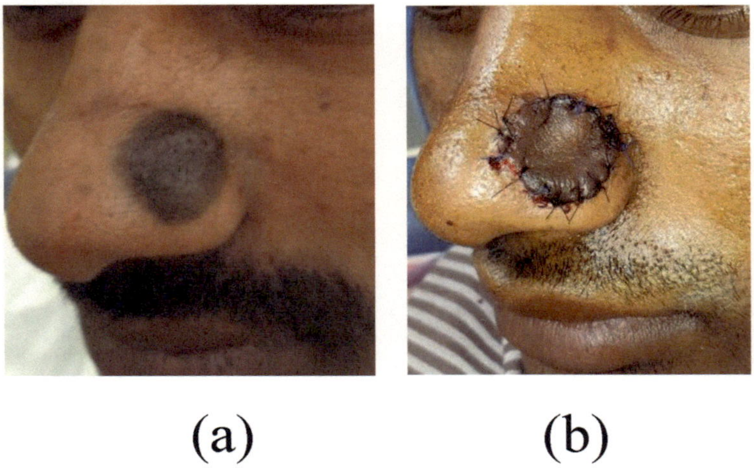

Figure 3.
(a) A case of melanocytic naevus. (b) Initial healing of Skin graft after bolster removal.

Tie over dressing involves downward pressure on the skin graft surface thereby adapting the skin graft well onto the recipient area thus eliminating the hematoma and seroma formation leading to good take of the skin graft. The principle of tie over dressing remains as simple as that.

Such a simple technique also is accountable for flipside issues inviting criticism. The downward pressure when it exceeds the capillary pressure, can cause graft damage. Prolonged intraoperative time and graft healing time, technique sensitive procedure, may hinder inspection and wound care in the postoperative period are other disadvantages. Also, no Randomized Control trials exist to prove the superiority of tie over technique over non tie over techniques [9].

3.2.2 Negative wound therapy

Negative wound therapy consists of application of gauze packs over the skin graft which is sealed by sticking an adhesive dressing. The dressing consists of a small fenestration that is connected to the vaccum regulator with the pressure maintained at 125 mm Hg.

Mohsin et al. concluded from their study that negative wound therapy has the following advantages.

- decreases the need for secondary coverage procedures.
- shortens the length of hospital stay.
- Early healing [10].

3.2.3 Non pressure dressings

Netscher and associates advocate moist non adherent gauze applied over the grafted site and is secured with self-adhering foam. Application and removal of the dressings are technically easy and it offers an even pressure over the grafted area [11].

Saltz and Bowles also advocate using Reston foam applied over Xenoform gauze as graft dressings [12]. Minami and colleagues acknowledge the usefulness of polyurethane dressings over the skin grafts as such dressings avoid the risks of pressure necrosis that is seen in tie over dressings [13].

Balakrishnan advocates the use of Lyofoam, which is applied over the graft directly. It is an inert, bacteriostatic, semipermeable polyurethane foam that enhances reepithelialization. Its inner surface is smooth and hydrophilic and outer surface is hydrophobic. Lyofoam is directly applied over the skin grafts and secured with staples [14].

3.2.4 Fibrin glue/octyl-2-cyanoacrylate ("super glue")

Fibrin sealant, two component material composed of fibrin and thrombin has been widely used as an adhesive for the skin graft ever since it got FDA approved. When applied at the skin edges it exhibits a remarkable adhesion property [15].

It has been advocated for its property of improving graft survival, reducing blood loss, hastening healing over large surface and thereby produces better results. A thin layer of fibrin glue significantly improves the graft take especially in mobile parts of the body [16].

3.2.5 Quilting

Quilting involves placing basing sutures on the surface of the graft thereby adapting it well to the recipient bed. Such quilting sutures are generally placed using absorbable ones. They are aimed at reducing the dead space in the graft that can lead to seroma formation.

In a study conducted by Yuhui Wu, the quilting sutures have been documented to reduce grade 2 and 3 seroma thereby improving the healing [17].

Other dressing materials are listed in the **Table 1.**

3.2.6 Tie over dressing vs. non tie over technique

Akhavani et al. and Dhillon et al. compared both these techniques to find out there is no statistically significant difference in graft take rate and infections. Even a study conducted by Yuki et al. in 266 patients also concluded the same [32–34].

S. no	Author	Dressing used
1	Johnson, Flemming and Avery [18]	staples with latex foam
2	Wolf and coworkers [19]	Rubber foam with staples
3	Smoot [20]	Staples and xenoform sandwich filled with cotton
4	Amir et al. [21]	Disposable syringes and silk threads
5	Cheng and colleagues [22]	Base of the IV infusion bottle and silk sutures
6	Vloemans and colleagues [23]	silicone rubber dressings
7	Sawada [24]	and silicone gel sheets
8	Renz BM [25]	rubber band stents
9	Ren J [26]	transparent gasbag tie-over dressings
10	Ward RS [27]	Coban self-adherent wrap
11	Grabski WJ [28]	thin hydrocolloid dressing
12	Watson SB [29] Balakrishanan C [30] Wells MD [31]	Assorted Silastic and foam dressings

Table 1.
Other dressing materials documented.

In our experience, the application of pressure over the skin graft becomes an optional entity and is sometimes dictated only by the anatomical area to be grafted. Any anatomical area that displays frequent movement that self-endangers the viability of the skin graft needs a Tie over dressing. Also an anatomical area where dead space creates the risk of seroma or hematoma collection compromising the adaptation of skin graft requires a tie over dressing for better adaptation. This again confirms the evidences that draw inconclusive evidences about the best type of skin graft fixation techniques.

In certain cases, absorbable sutures are preferred over the silk sutures as the silk gets buried while the bolster is removed when the healing is complete. Although our experience with cyanoacrylate glue is limited, the idea of applying any material other than autogenous entities had always raised concerns for the fear of it instilling hypersensitivity reactions.

3.3 Challenging anatomical areas for skin graft fixation

The advances in the ablative surgical techniques have only left with more complexities for the reconstruction procedures. The necessity and the radical nature of oncologic resections carried out in the head and neck areas demand meticulous reconstructive measures that make them challenging [35].

3.3.1 Reconstruction of the sinus cavities

Post resection, the skin graft is secured with sutures in the sinus lining and available cancellous bone surfaces. The sinus is stuffed with petrolatum gauze that would offer even pressure over the skin graft surface. One of the ends of the gauze is seen jetting out through orifices created intraorally or at the face near the floor of the orbit. After the healing, the gauze is gently removed out through the orifices. The remaining orifice defects are addressed prosthetically.

3.3.2 Reconstruction of alveolus

The alveolar bone is trimmed to make the cancellous bone exposed. The skin graft margins are adapted perfectly over the cancellous bone surface and adjacent soft tissue. Sutures are placed if possible. Acrylic stent dressing is placed over the gauze dressing.

In mandible, the acrylic is secured in situ by circum mandibular wiring. In maxilla, the acrylic stent is secured by peralveolar wiring or lateral suspension wiring.

3.3.3 Reconstruction of floor of mouth

The skin graft adaptation and securing is carried out by help of sutures. The gauze foam dressing that is applied over the graft is secured with suture ties that run to the supra hyoid region where it is anchored.

3.3.4 Reconstruction of palate

Palatal skin graft fixation requires construction of a Hawley's appliance with a palatal extension that would fill in the defect. This acrylic stent is fabricated preoperatively and is applied over the palatal skin graft (**Figure 4a** and **b**).

3.3.5 Reconstruction of tongue

The tongue is an extremely mobile organ where the skin graft fixation becomes very difficult. The grafted site is covered with foam dressing. The tongue is then compressed into the floor of the mouth by the fixation of a plate lined with foam-rubber sponge. The plate in turn is anchored to the teeth using wires or with circummandibular wiring if edentulous.

Tongue physiotherapy is carried out post healing to prevent fibrosis.

3.3.6 Reconstruction of larynx

After the appropriate portions of the laryngeal structures have been excised, inclusive of the homolateral laryngeal tissues and frequently passes beyond the anterior commissure or posterior commissure to the opposite cord, the graft is fitted

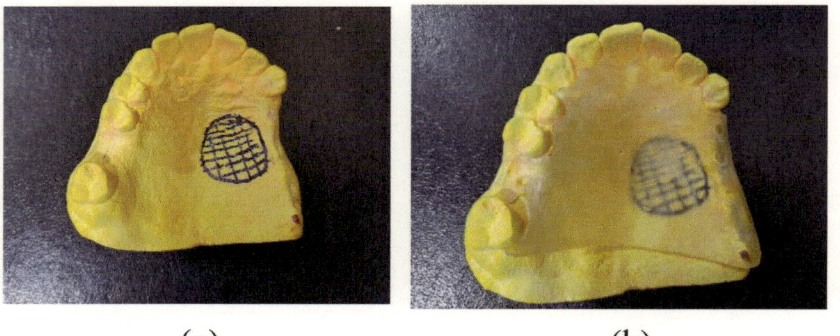

(a) (b)

Figure 4.
(a) Model with diagrammatic presentation of extent of the defect. (b) Acrylic stent.

to the outside of a modeled tantalum wire-mesh or plastic framework and carefully sutured into position. The position is maintained by a stent that avoids stenosis due to contraction.

4. Conclusion

In conclusion, the skin graft techniques and dressings are few in number for consideration and have their own indications, merits and demerits. Functionally all the fixation techniques when done well and proper serve the healing of the graft well. No technique rules over the other with better benefits. Evidence of comparison of the fixation techniques also prove the same till date. Future is foreseen to develop newer techniques for graft fixation and dressings and more evidence based comparison for arriving at better conclusions.

Acknowledgements

Dr.Manjunath N.M. MDS, M Phil,FAM, FAOCMF Consultant Oral and Maxillofacial Surgeon, Director of Dew Dental and maxillofacial Center, Bangalore, Karnataka. Dr.Venkatasubramanian MCh Plastic Surgery, pudhukottai, Tamil nadu. Dr.Murali Manivannan, MCh.,MRCS (Edin), DNB, Consultant Vascular Surgeon, Thanjavur Medical college and Hospital, Thanjavur, Tamil nadu.

Conflict of interest

The authors declare no conflict of interest.

Notes/thanks/other declarations

I extend my sincere thanks and gratitude to Dr. Gauthami Sundar and Dr. Rajaram for the Literature support. My deep sense of gratitude to Dr. Murali Manivannan for the timely contributions for the chapter.

Author details

Sundaram Ravanasamudram Rajaram[1]* and Gauthami Sundar[2]

1 University of Science and Technology, Fujairah, United Arab Emirates

2 Dr.Rajaram's Dental Surgery, Thanjavur, India

*Address all correspondence to: sundarum88@gmail.com

References

[1] Chick LR. Brief history and biology of skin grafting. Ann Plast Surg 1988;21:358-365.

[2] Davis JS. Address of the President: The Story of Plastic Surgery. Ann Surg 1941;113:641-656.

[3] HaywardL. Surgicalneedles, ancient and modern.Transactions of the Institute of British Surgical Technicians1961;1:18.4 Druitt R. The Surgeon's Vademecum, 8th edition.

[4] Dresdale A, Rose EA, Jeevanandam V, Reemtsma K, Bowman FO, Malm JR. Preparation of fibrin glue from single-donor fresh-frozen plasma. Surgery. 1985 Jun; 97 (6):750-755. PMID: 3873716.

[5] Bergel S (1909) Uber wirkungen des fibrins. Dtsch Med Wochenschr 35:633

[6] Burleson R, Eiseman B: Nature of the bond between partial-thickness skin and wound granulations. Am Surg 177:181, 1973. 84.

[7] Tavis MJ, Thornton JW, Harney JH, et al: Graft adherence to de-epithelialized surfaces: a comparative study. Ann Surg 184:594, 1976

[8] Han HH, Jun D, Moon SH, Kang IS, Kim MC. Fixation of split-thickness skin graft using fast-clotting fibrin glue containing undiluted high-concentration thrombin or sutures: a comparison study. Springerplus. 2016;5(1):1902

[9] Kromka W, Cameron M, Fathi R. Tie-over bolster dressings vs basting sutures for the closure of full-thickness skin grafts: A review of the literature. J Cutan Med Surg. 2018;22:602-606.

[10] Mohsin M, Zargar HR, Wani AH, Zaroo MI, Baba PUF, Bashir SA, Rasool A, Bijli AH. Role of customised negative-pressure wound therapy in the integration of split-thickness skin grafts: A randomised control study. Indian J Plast Surg. 2017 Jan-Apr;50(1):43-49.

[11] Netscher DT, Marchi M, Wigoda P: A method for optimizing skin graft healing and outcome of wounds of the penile shaft and scrotum. Ann Plast Surg 31:447, 1993.

[12] Saltz R, Bowles BJ: Reston: an alternate method of skin graft fixation (letter). Plast Reconstr Surg 99:601, 1997

[13] Minami RT,Holderness H, Vistnes LM. A tie over dressing with polyurethane foam. Plast Reconstr Surg 1973;52:672

[14] Balakrishnan C: Dressing for skin grafts of the penis (letter). Plast Reconstr Surg 95:208, 1995

[15] William D. Spotnitz. Fibrin Sealant: Past, Present, and Future: A Brief Review. World J Surg (2010) 34:632-634 DOI 10.1007/s00268-009-0252-7

[16] Currie LJ, Sharpe JR, Martin R: The use of fibrin glue in skin grafts and tissue-engineered skin replacements: a review. Plast Reconstr Surg 108:1713, 2001.

[17] Wu, Y., Wang, S., Hai, J. *et al.* Quilting suture is better than conventional suture with drain in preventing seroma formation at pectoral area after mastectomy. BMC Surg 20, 65 (2020). https://doi.org/10.1186/s12893-020-00725-8

[18] Johnson PA, Fleming K, Avery CME: Latex foam and staple fixation of skin grafts. Br J Oral Maxillofac Surg 36:141, 1998.

[19] Wolf Y, Kalish E, Badani E, et al: Rubber foam and staples: do they secure

skin grafts? A model analysis and proposal of pressure enhancement techniques. Ann Plast Surg 40:149, 1998.

[20] Smoot EC: A rapid method for splinting skin grafts and securing wound dressings (letter). Plast Reconstr Surg 100:1622, 1997.

[21] Amir A, Sagi A, Fliss DM, Rosenberg L: A simple, rapid, reproducible tie-over dressing. Plast Reconstr Surg 98:1092, 1996.

[22] Cheng LC, Lim TC, Tan WTL: A simple tie-over dressing (letter). Plast Reconstr Surg 101:246, 1998.

[23] Vloemans AFPM, Kreis RW: Fixation of skin grafts with a new silicone rubber dressing (Mepitel). Scand J Plast Reconstr Surg 28:75, 1994.

[24] Sawada Y, Yotsuyanagi T, Ara M, Sone K: Experiences using silicone gel tie-over dressings following skin grafting. Burns 16:353, 1990.

[25] Renz BM, Stout M, Sherman R: Rubberband stents for skin grafts: how I do it. Am Surg 60:707, 1994.

[26] Ren J, Yiang OJ, Deng B, Yiang YN: Transparent gasbag tieover for persistent pressure and inspection in free skin grafting. Plast Reconstr Surg 95:396, 1995.

[27] Ward RS, Reddy R, Brockway C, et al: Uses of Coban selfadherent wrap in management of postburn hand grafts: case reports. J Burn Care Rehabil 15:364, 1994.

[28] Grabski WJ, Giandoni MB, Anderson LL: Surgical pearl: hydrocolloid dressings for full-thickness skin grafts. J Am Acad Dermatol 32:273, 1995.

[29] Watson SB, Miller JG: Optimizing skin graft take in children's hand burns—the use of Silastic foam dressings. Burns 19:519, 1993.

[30] Balakrishnan C: Simple method of applying pressure to skin grafts of neck with foam dressing and staples. J Burn Care Rehabil 15:432, 1994.

[31] Wells MD, Kirn DS: A new method of skin-graft stabilization: the Reston technique. Ann Plast Surg 34:554, 1995.

[32] Akhavani MA, McKinnell T, Kang NV. Quilting of full thickness grafts in the hand. J Plast Reconstr Aesthet Surg. 2010;63(9):1534-1537.

[33] Dhillon M, Carter CP, Morrison J, Hislop WS, Currie WJ. A comparison of skin graft success in the head & neck with and without the use of a pressure dressing. J Maxillofac Oral Surg. 2015;14(2):240-242.

[34] Yuki, A., Takenouchi, T., Takatsuka, S., Fujikawa, H. and Abe, R. (2017), Investigating the use of tie-over dressing after skin grafting. J Dermatol, 44: 1317-1319. https://doi.org/10.1111/1346-8138.13916

[35] John J. C. Free skin grafting in the sinus, Oral, and Pharyngeal areas in Radical surgery of the Head and Neck, Head and Neck Department of the Pack Medical Group and the Surgical Service OE St. Vincent's Hospital, New York, New York. Dec 5, 1953.

Chapter 6

Procurement and Use of Cryopreserved Total Skin Allograft in Complex Wounds

Marcelo Fonseca, Aldo Cañete, Dino Ibaceta, Catalina Buchroithner, Florencia Disi and Juan Olivares

Abstract

Cryopreserved total skin allografts are a new therapeutic alternative for the management of complex wounds. Their properties allow them to be classified as a temporary coverage for some patients and as definitive in others. And they can be an alternative option to the use of dermal regeneration templates.

Keywords: skin allograft, biological dressings, wound healing, skin substitutes, dermal regenerators

1. Introduction

Historically, choosing the therapeutic options for the management of complex wounds was based on the concept of the "reconstructive ladder", in which reconstructive methods were ranked by complexity and the simplest options capable of solving the problem had to be chosen. The latter has evolved over time, with the emergence of the "reconstructive elevator concept", where a surgeon can ascend directly to the appropriate level in order to obtain the best qualified reconstruction, and due to the need of incorporating new advances in wound healing management into the "reconstructive ladder" [1, 2].

The use of skin allografts (SA) for wound coverage began during the 19th century. Currently occupy a predominant place within the temporary coverage techniques, especially in burn patients, with little residual skin capital, and with extensive clinical experience in other pathologies [3–7]. SA provide a physiological lining to control the hydro electrolyte losses, reduce the pain and infection risk and improve local bed conditions by promoting angiogenesis and the maturation of the underlying granulation tissue [8, 9]. However, due to immunological processes, they are usually rejected after 10–12 days and may eventually be a vector for infectious diseases [10, 11].

Most of the SA come from cadaveric donor; are harvested as partial skin grafts (**Figure 1A**) with a dermatome and are preserved using glycerol at high concentrations, causing cellular death with the obtention of non-viable tissues [12, 13].

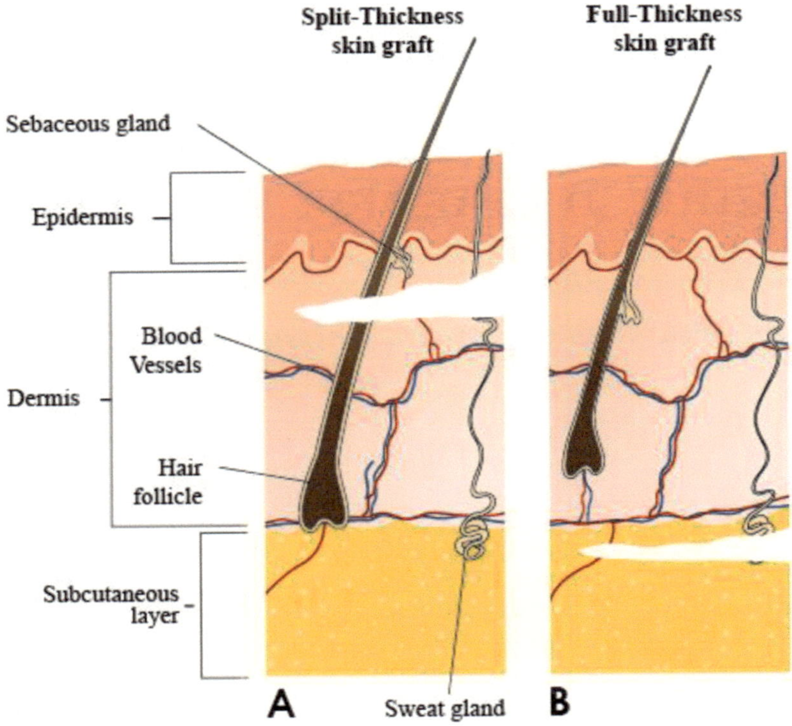

Figure 1.
A. Split-thickness skin graft B. Total skin allografts.

2. Cryopreserved total skin allografts

2.1 Background

The low rate of human organ and tissue donation and the cultural and religious restrictions for the use of cadaveric tissues in certain countries, have opened the door to the pursuit of other sources of SA, particularly in patients who underwent body contouring surgeries (abdominoplasty, reductive mammoplasty), either for esthetic or reconstructive reasons. This allows the entire resected flap to be procured, allowing the obtention of total skin allografts (TSA) (**Figure 1B**) [14–17].

2.2 Tissue production

The process of obtaining TSA is initiated with the invitation of patients who are candidates for body contouring surgeries to participate in the donation of the redundant fatty skin flap, which would otherwise be a waste product. This represents the first difference with SA obtained from corpses, the TSA are obtained from living donors. Donors are submitted under a health survey (**Table 1**), the absence of exclusion criteria is verified (**Table 2**) and routine examinations for tissue donation are performed (**Table 3**). All the above is assessed to guarantee the microbiological safety of the tissues, which is mainly based on the selection of the donor, permitting the rejection of infections or any biological agent that could cause diseases in the recipient [18].

	YES	NO
Are you in good health today?		
Are you in generally good health?		
Did you sleep at least 5 hours?		
Have you drunk alcohol in the last 12 hours?		
Have you donated blood in the last year?		
Have you been told by a health professional that you cannot donate blood?		
Have you been to another doctor's office in the last 6 months?		
Have you had a dental procedure over the last week?		
Have you been hospitalized or operated during the last 6 months?		
Have you received any transfusion in the last 12 months?		
Have you had any blood tests in the last 12 months?		
Do you have or have had any heart, lung, kidney or thyroid disease, hypertension, diabetes mellitus, bleeding tendency or other illness?		
Are you taking any medication on a regular basis in the last 6 months?		
Have you taken aspirin or anti-inflammatory drugs in the last 3 days?		
Have you had any injections or vaccinations in the last 4 days?		
Have you had diarrhea in the last 7 days?		
Have you ever had cancer?		
Do you have a history of epilepsy, seizures or fainting?		
Do you have or had hepatitis or have you turned yellow?		
Have you had any tissue transplants or grafts?		
Have you received growth hormone treatment before 1985?		
Do you have a family history of Creutzfeldt-Jakob disease?		
Do you or your family have a history of dementia, Alzheimer's, Parkinson's, Multiple Sclerosis or another degenerative disease?		
Do you or your family have a history of Chagas disease?		
Have you had Malaria, Dengue fever or unexplained fever during or after a trip outside the country?		
Have you traveled outside the country in the last 3 years; if yes, where?		
Have you had any tattoo, piercing, acupuncture or accidental needle stick or bloody syringe in the last 6 months?		
Have you tried any type of drug such as marijuana, cocaine, cocaine paste or other; if yes, which ones and when?		
Have you used illegal injectable or inhalant drugs over the last 12 months?		
Have you had sexual intercourse with anyone who has ever injected drugs?		
Have you had sexually transmitted diseases such as Syphilis, Gonorrhea or other in the last 12 months?		
Have you had more than one sexual partner in the last 12 months?		
Have you had sexual intercourse with a new partner in the last 6 months?		
Have you had sexual contact with persons with Hepatitis, HIV or HTLV in the last 12 months?		
Have you paid or received money, drugs, or anything else for sex in the last 12 months?		
Have you been exposed to the risk of becoming infected with the AIDS virus?		

	YES	NO
Are you donating tissue so that you can be tested for AIDS?		
Have you been offered money to donate your tissue?		

HIV: human immunodeficiency virus; HTLV: human T-lymphotropic virus; AIDS: Acquired immunodeficiency syndrome.

Table 1.
Living tissue donor questionnaire.

It is important to mention that patients submitted to bariatric surgery with a secondary weight loss, have cutaneous structure and histological changes. Including a lower fibroblast and elastin concentration and collagen fiber organization, sites of chronic inflammation, sebaceous glands infections and metalloproteinases levels similar to the skin of patients with cancer and burns. Therefore, it is expected that the quality of TSAs from this group of patients will be lower [19, 20]. After the donor selection, the process is divided into 10 stages: 1) surgical procedure/body contouring surgery, 2) procurement itself, 3) packaging and identification, 4) storage, 5) transport to the processing center, 6) processing, 7) cryopreservation/quarantine, 8) validation, release, records, 9) transfer and 10) clinical use. All of the above must be within the framework of an organ and tissue donation program that permits the generation and guarantee products of high: biological quality, sanitary safety and therapeutic value [21].

2.2.1 Surgical procedure/body contouring surgery

The skin processing is performed in the operating room, at the same time as the body contouring surgery, with all asepsis and antisepsis measures, under general anesthesia and by the same surgical team. After the redundant skin marking and the adipose skin flap dissection, the resection of the flap is performed. Subsequently, two teams are formed: one finishes the body contouring surgery and the other, on a separate surgical table, performs the skin procurement.

2.2.2 Skin treatment

The dissected adipose skin flap is placed on a separate operating table. Total skin procurement (including dermis) is performed, removing the fat from the deeper dermis with scissors (**Figure 2**). Tissue samples (3) are also taken for current (aerobic), anaerobic and fungal culture. The procured skin is placed in a sterile container with 500 cc of physiological saline solution with 1 g of Cloxacillin and 80 mg of Gentamicin, hermetically closed, making sure the skin is completely submerged. This process of the allograft obtention gives the second distinctive characteristic to the TSAs: they are total skin allografts.

2.2.3 Packaging and skin identification

The vials containing the skin are stored in double sterile bags of at least 90 microns. Each vial is hermetically sealed, removing as much air as possible, and labeled with the tissue code and the date and time of processing.

2.2.4 Skin storage

The skin is transferred from the operating room to a temporary storage place in a refrigeration unit, in order to maintain the temperature between 2 and 8°C.

Exclusion criteria:

a. For infectious diseases
   - Patients with history or carriers of HIV/AIDS.
   - Patients with a history of Hepatitis B or C.
   - Patients with a history of active Tuberculosis.
   - Patients diagnosed with Syphilis or positive VDRL.
   - Patients diagnosed with HTLV I and II.
   - Patients diagnosed with Chagas disease.
   - Patients with diagnosis of Rabies, Congenital Rubella and Malaria.
   - Patients diagnosed with untreated bacterial or fungal endocarditis.

b. For central nervous system diseases
   - Degenerative diseases
     a. Any type or manifestation of Dementia.
     b. Alzheimer's disease.
     c. Parkinson's disease.
     d. Multiple sclerosis.
     e. Creutzfeldt-Jakob disease.
   - Infectious diseases
     a. Bacterial encephalitis.
     b. Viral, fungal or parasitic meningitis.
     c. Bacterial meningitis.
     d. Progressive multifocal leukoencephalopathy.
     e. Subacute sclerosing panencephalitis.
     f. Active viral encephalitis or encephalitis of unknown cause.
     g. Fungal or parasitic encephalitis.

c. For presence of cancer and/or tumors
   - History of neoplasia except for cervical uterine cancer in situ.
   - Lymphadenopathy for more than one month.
   - Lymphomas, lymphosarcomas
   - Leukemias.
   - Metastasis of primary or secondary malignant tumors (lung, breast, cervical, colon, prostate, squamous cell, melanomas, lymphomas, leukemias, central nervous system, among others).

d. Other pathologies
   - Patients who have been treated with growth hormone.
   - Patients with Hemophilia.
   - Patients carriers of autoimmune diseases or Mesenchymopathies such as Rheumatoid Arthritis, Systemic Lupus Erythematosus.
   - Patients who have been treated with prolonged corticosteroid therapy.
   - Any suspicious skin alteration.

e. Behavioral:
   - Unsafe sexual behavior.
   - Drug abuse (including intravenous, intramuscular and subcutaneous).
   - Commercial sex workers.
   - Inmates.
   - Individuals with tattoos, (or) body piercing performed in the last 6 months.
   - Individuals from whom no history of sexual behavior can be collected.

f. Specific skin criteria:
   - Skin contaminated by toxins.
   - Pyoderma.
   - Any skin lesion: infectious, traumatic or vascular.
   - Psoriasis.
   - Epidermolysis bullosa.
   - Loxocelism.
   - Structurally damaged skin (due to autoimmune or collagen diseases).

HIV: human immunodeficiency virus; HTLV: human T-lymphotropic virus; AIDS: Acquired immunodeficiency syndrome; VDRL: Venereral Disease Research Laboratory.

Table 2.
Exclusion criteria for skin donation.

1. Hepatitis B surface antigen.
2. Antibodies against Hepatitis C.
3. Antibodies against HIV.
4. VDRL
5. HTLV I and II.
6. Chagas.
7. Cultures intraoperative
    - Standard culture (aerobic)
    - Anaerobic culture
    - Mycotic culture.

HIV: human immunodeficiency virus; HTLV: human T-lymphotropic virus; VDRL: Venereral Disease Research Laboratory.

Table 3.
Laboratory tests.

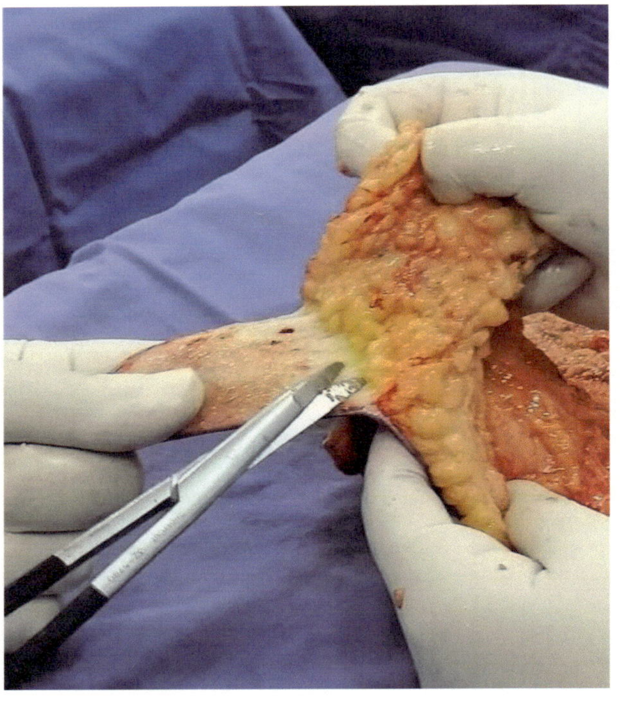

Figure 2.
Procurement of total skin with scissors from redundant adipose skin flap.

2.2.5 Skin transportation

The skin is sent for processing, in our particular case, to the National Tissue Bank (NTB), always within 36 hours from harvesting, assuring the container maintains a temperature between 2 and 8°C.

2.2.6 Processing

The TSAs are prepared in the NBT as implants, following two stages: In the first one, the measurement of the flap is conducted, performing cuts in segments of different sizes according to the request; for example, in an average abdominoplasty, approximately 300 cm^2 of useful surface are obtained.

Subsequently, a revision of the shaving, washing cycles (to reduce the microbial load), obtention of sample number 2 for cultures (the first one was intraoperative) and immersion in cryopreservative solution for 1 hour are performed. In the second stage, the preparation, cutting, measurement, packaging and labeling of each obtained flap is conducted. Samples number 3 and 4 are taken for culture, which are performed during the packaging stage. Finally, a 5th sample is taken, also for culture, as a backup.

2.2.7 Cryopreservation and quarantine

Cryopreservation freezes the TSAs in the presence of a cryoprotectant (10% glycerol), which prevents the crystallization effects while maintaining viability over time after freezing. Viability being understood as the capacity of a biological unit to remain alive. The cryopreserved total skin allograft (CTSA) is kept frozen at −80°C awaiting the results of serial cultures until irradiation. The latter is performed with a dose of 25 to 28 kGy, in dry ice to maintain the cold chain, being a complementary procedure for tissue sterilization. The viability of the tissues obtained gives the third distinctive characteristic to CTSAs, which is fundamental for the clinical results [22, 23].

2.2.8 Validation, release and records

An adequate quality management system requires having a dossier or record of each tissue processed, which allows the evaluation of each of the steps from the generation to the implantation of the CTSAs in the recipient, permitting the monitorization and traceability. Once the donation, procurement and processing procedures have been reviewed and the microbiological results have been verified, the tissues are released for clinical use.

2.2.9 Transportation

Following the tissue release, they are transferred for clinical use on dry ice, maintaining the cold chain (−80°C).

2.2.10 Clinical use

In the preoperative period, the size of the defect to be covered should be calculated in order to choose the CTSAs. The CTSAs should be washed 3 times with warm saline (no more than 40°C) to remove cryoprotectants. The wound bed is prepared by resection of necrotic, devitalized tissues and areas with granulation disorder. The CTSAs is fixed with stitches and/or brackets associated with negative pressure therapy [24].

3. Clinic

The CTSA has an initial attachment similar to an autologous skin graft, to later evolve towards rejection, at 21 days average, which is clinically evidenced by coloration change and the formation of a superficial necrotic eschar. When the latter is removed, it exposes vital tissue adhered to the host (**Figure 3**).

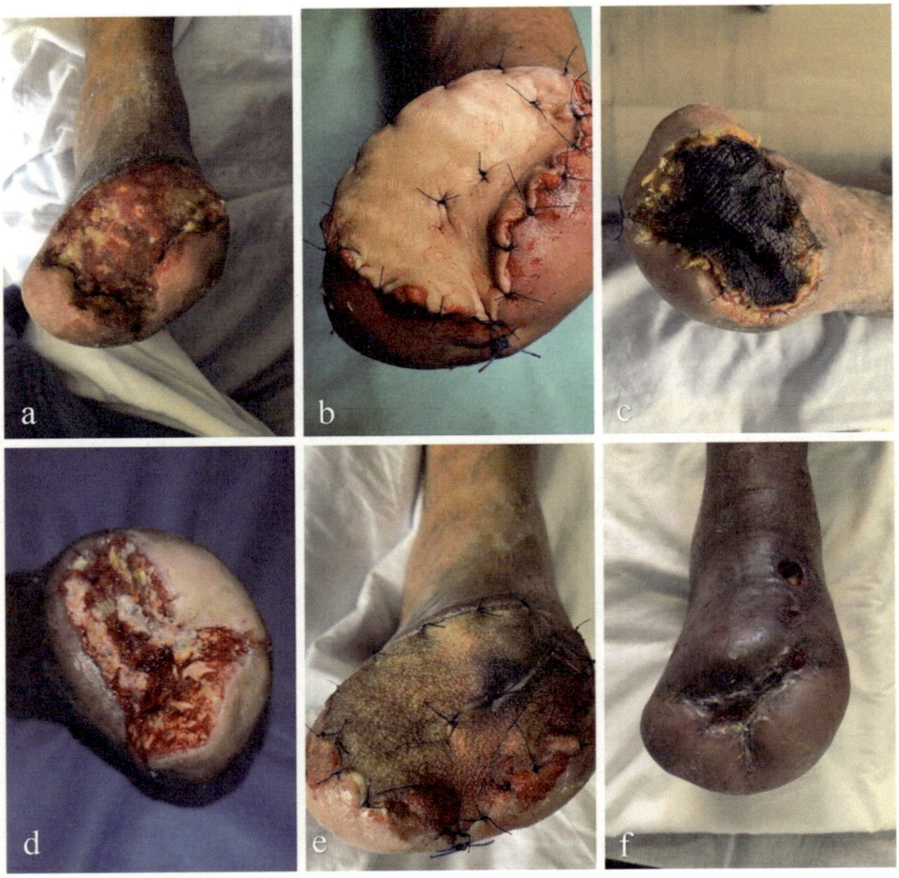

Figure 3.
Diabetic patient, 68 years old, with flap necrosis after transmetarsal amputation. a. Coverage deficit with bone exposure associated with disordered granulatory tissue. b. Coverage with CTASs. c. Evolution CTASs after 28 days. d. Receiving bed after escharectomy of superficial part of CTASs. e. Partial skin autograft, result at day 7, which was subsequently lost in its entirety and managed with advanced healing. f. Result: 4 months after initial surgery.

This is evidenced histologically in the CTSAs by necrosis foci with infiltration mainly of nuclear polymorphs (**Figure 4a**) and in the recipient bed by the presence of an interface rich in fibroblasts and neoformation vessels (**Figure 4b**).

This interface or neo-dermis is also visualized with imaging studies; in magnetic resonance imaging (MRI) CTSAs can be seen with a superficial non-catching component and a deep component that is enhanced by the contrast medium, similar to the vascularized dermis (**Figure 5**) [25]. For SA, it had already been described that some elements of the dermis, mainly fibroblasts, could be permanently integrated into the host, with exceptional situations of complete attachment and absence of rejection of the SA. The most mediatic case involved Sir Winston Churchill, who during the Nile War, donated skin and it was grafted to a wounded comrade and "remains there to this day and has lasted well in many ways. Myself, keep the scar as a souvenir." [26–28].

CTSAs maintain the entire donor dermis, which participates in the proliferation of a neo-dermis rich in fibroblasts and neoforming vessels, also acting as a scaffold and a biological inducer in the wound bed. CTSAs have been shown in xenograft models to promote angiogenesis and type 1 collagen production without eliciting a significant fibrotic response [29]. Rejection of the CTSAs should not be interpreted

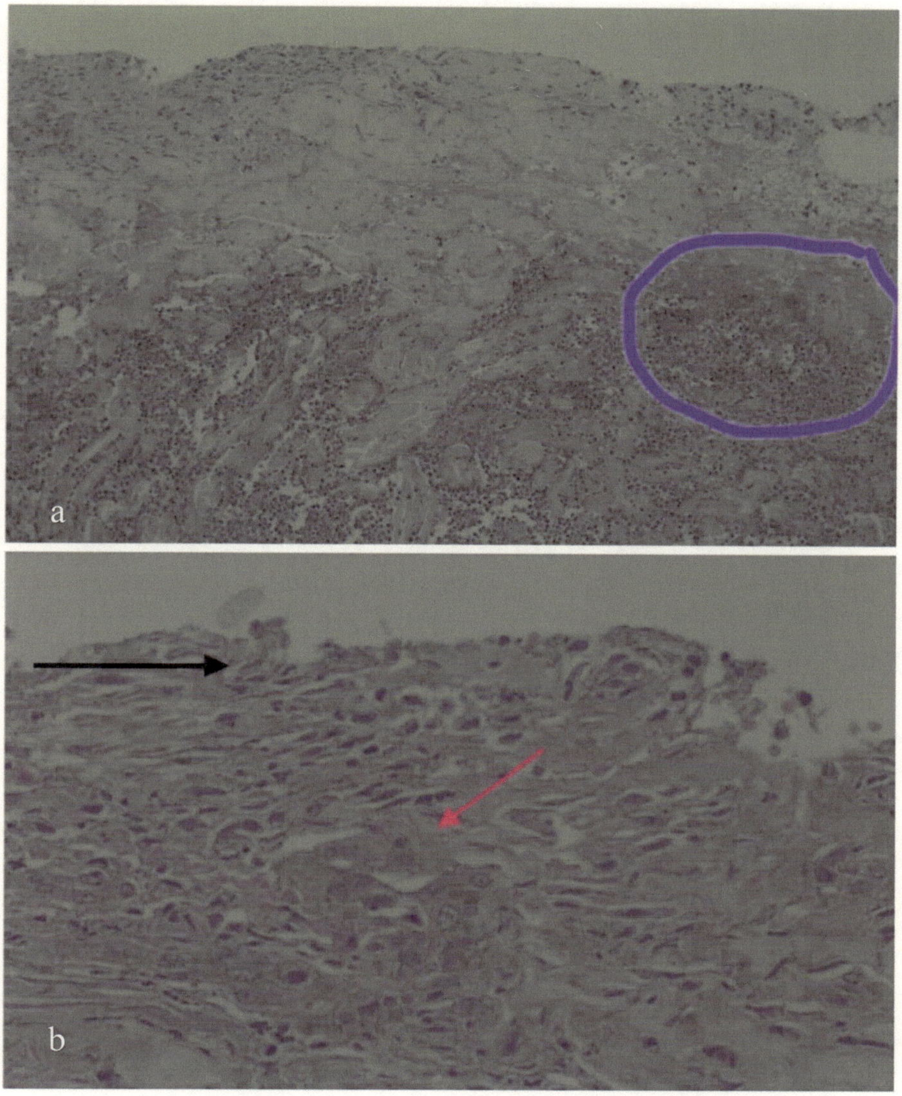

Figure 4.
a. Histology. Hematoxylin/eosin stain. CTSAs at the time of escharectomy (21 days). Circled are shows infiltration of nuclear polymorphs, necrosis areas. b. Post-CTSAs receptor bed. Black arrow: Fibroblasts, red arrow: Neoformation vessels.

as a therapeutic failure, but as a stage of what we have called intermediate coverage. Since part of the CTSAs is lost and part adheres to the recipient bed, obtaining an interface of neodermis allows the completion of the definitive coverage with an autograft and a complete healing by second intention. This also produces a secondary contraction of the wound, reducing size of the defect.

The increased survival of seriously burnt patients with severe sequels, mainly due to the limited contribution of the autologous partial skin graft dermis and second intention scarring of the burnt skin, was the main motive for the dermal matrix development. Currently, available dermal substitutes (biologic, synthetic or biosynthetic origin) are fundamentally used as a scaffolding or biocompatible structural support, that is colonized by the patient's cells in order to form a neodermis, which is practically identic in structure as the receipt's dermis [30–34].

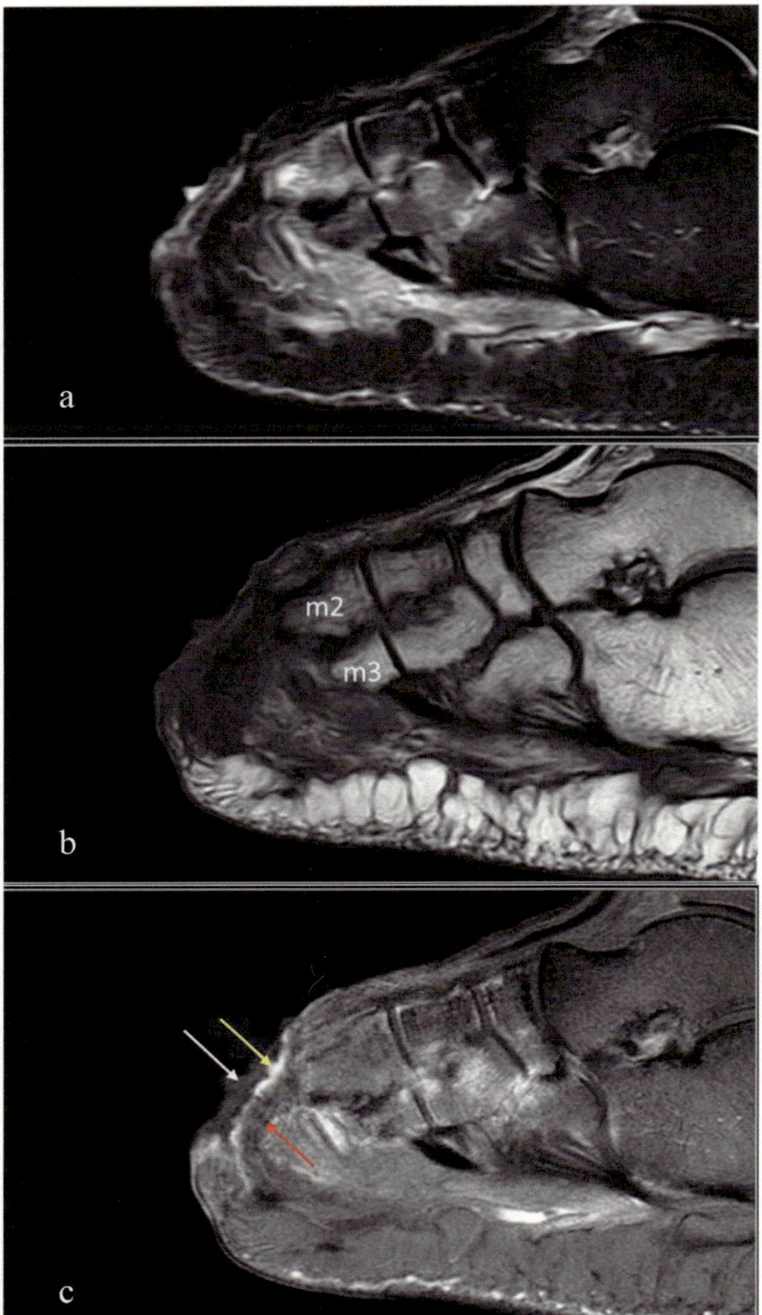

Figure 5.
Magnetic resonance images of the foot in the sagittal plane enhanced in STIR -short tau inversion recovery- (a), T1 (b) and T1 with fat saturation and contrast medium (c), showing the graft with a superficial non-capturing component (white arrow) and a deep component that enhances with the contrast medium (yellow arrow) similar to the vascularized dermis. Between the latter and the bone tissue, there is low signal material with discrete enhancement (red arrow). (m2: Second metatarsal; m3: Third metatarsal).

It is important to emphasize that dermal regeneration templates share various advantages with CTSAs, including: a) immediate wound closure, thus avoiding fluid loss and restoring the functional barrier of the skin, b) coverage of structures such as bone, cartilage and tendons and c) better scar quality and elasticity. But they differ mainly in the high cost of dermal regeneration templates, which is the main reason for their limited use in clinical practice, and the fact that they necessarily

Patient	Age	Genre	Diagnosis	Evolution
1	68 Y	Masc	Diabetic foot. Transmetatarsal amputation	Surgical debridement / bone resection / CTSA / Scarectomy / Split-thickness skin graft / graft loss / Advanced wound healing / **Figure 3**.
2	26 Y	Masc	Complex wound of the leg	Surgical debridement / CTSA / Advanced wound healing / Complete healing and closure
3*	53 Y	Fem	Relapsing Dermatofibrosarcoma of the scalp	Tumor resection / Skull Fenestration / CTSA / Advanced wound healing. **Figure 6**.
4	55 Y	Masc	Diabetic foot. Transmetatarsal amputation	Surgical debridement / CTSA / Scarectomy / Split-thickness skin graft / Loss of follow-up
5	70 Y	Masc	Abdominal sepsis. Open abdomen	Complicated inguinal hernia / abdominal sepsis / multi-organ failure / contained laparostomy, CTSA / clinical improvement/ extubation / Death due to pneumonia
6*	2 M	Masc	Premature. Necrotizing enterocolitis. Contained laparostomy.	Premature 30 weeks / Dysfunctionalisation of intestinal transit / evisceration (2 occasions) / Contained laparostomy / CTSA / Para-ostomal hernia and inguinal hernia. Periostomal and inguinal hernioplasty. **Figure 7**.
7	60 Y	Masc	Diabetic foot	Surgical debridement / scarectomy / CTSA / Split-thickness skin graft / 90% success / Loss of follow-up
8	49 Y	Masc	Diabetic foot	Surgical debridement / scarectomy / CTSA / Loss of follow-up
9	57 Y	Masc	Skin stripping of the leg	Scarectomy / CTSA / Split-thickness skin graft / 100% success.
10*	3 M	Masc	Premature. Necrotizing enterocolitis. Contained laparostomy.	Premature 30 weeks / CTSA replacement / Abdominal wall continent / Second intention healing. **Figure 7**.
11*	53 Y	Fem	Relapsing Dermatofibrosarcoma of the scalp	CTSA replacement in the central área / No autologous graft due to absence of neodermis in central area (initial bone wax in this area). **Figure 6**.
12	75 Y	Masc	Melanoma of the cheek	Melanoma (biopsy confirmed) resection. Local flap reconstruction.
13	83 Y	Masc	Melanoma of the forearm	Melanoma resection. Staging in process.
14	56 Y	Masc	Diabetic foot	Surgical debridement / bone resection / CTSA / Scarectomy / Split-thickness skin graft / Advanced wound healing / complete wound closure
15	31 Y	Fem	Necrotizing fasciitis of the forearm	Surgical debridement / CTSA / Awaiting progress for skin autografting.

*Years (Y), Months (M), Femenine (Fem), Masculine (Masc), CTSA: Cryopreserved total skin allograft. * Patient undergoing two interventions with cryopreserved total skin allograft.*

Table 4.
Clinical experience. Summary.

require a second time for skin autografting. Regarding the latter is that CTSAs can be used as an alternative to dermal regeneration templates [35, 36].

4. Clinical experience

Our clinical experience was initiated on August 1st, 2020 and persists to the date. Mainly following the pursuit of cutaneous coverages for seriously burnt patients, given the lack of dermal regeneration matrix since their high cost and limited availability. The latter is supported by the disposal of concomitant residual abdominal skin grafts following abdominoplasty surgeries. The donor sample was constituted by fourteen female patients, of 31 to 55 years with an average age of 40 years. The receipt sample was composed by 13 patients (two patients underwent two surgical procedures), ages ranging from 2 months to 83 years. With the following diagnosis: Diabetic foot (5), contained laparostomy (2) complex extremities wounds (3), relapsed scalp sarcoma (1) and melanoma (2) [37]. Clinical evolution is summarized in **Table 4**.

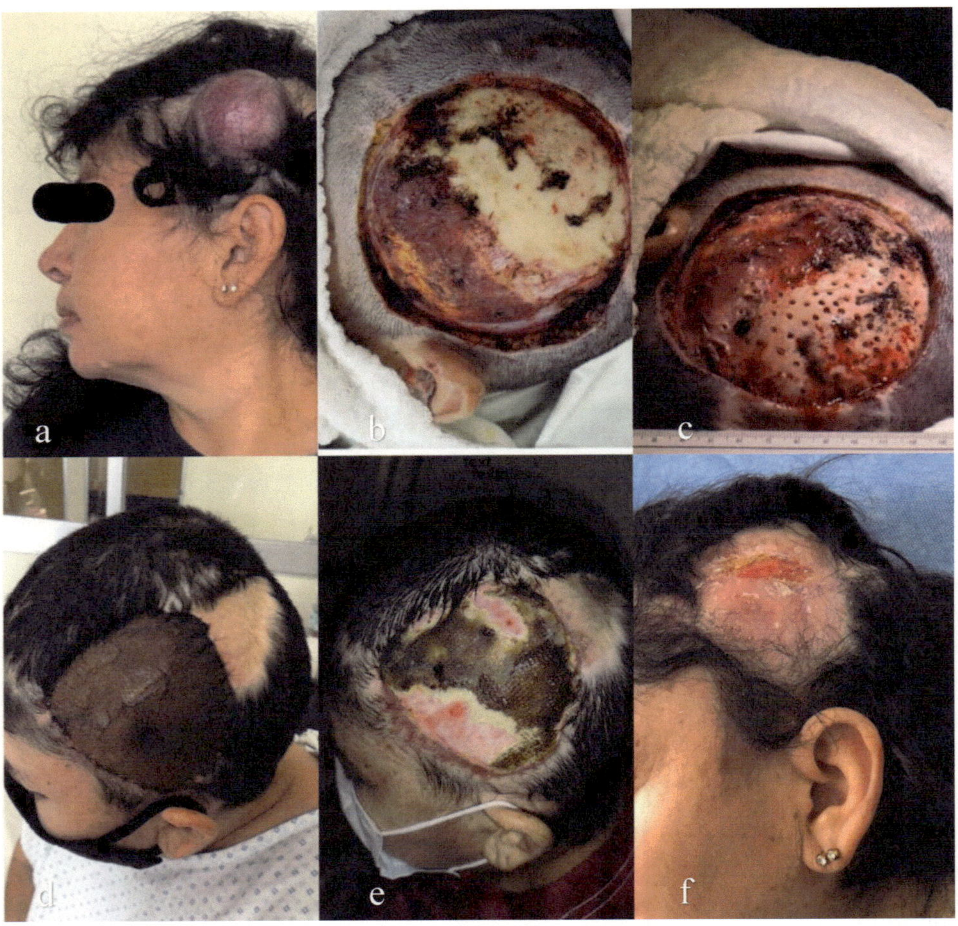

Figure 6.
Female patient, 53 years old. With a history of dermatosarcoma of the scalp. With resection and subsequent reconstruction with local flaps and partial skin grafts. Tumour recurrence. a. Dermatosarcoma of the scalp. b. Defect of coverage post resection. c. Fenestration of the skull. d. CTSA 30 days. e. CTSA 60 days f. CTSA 150 days, completely healed wound by second intention.

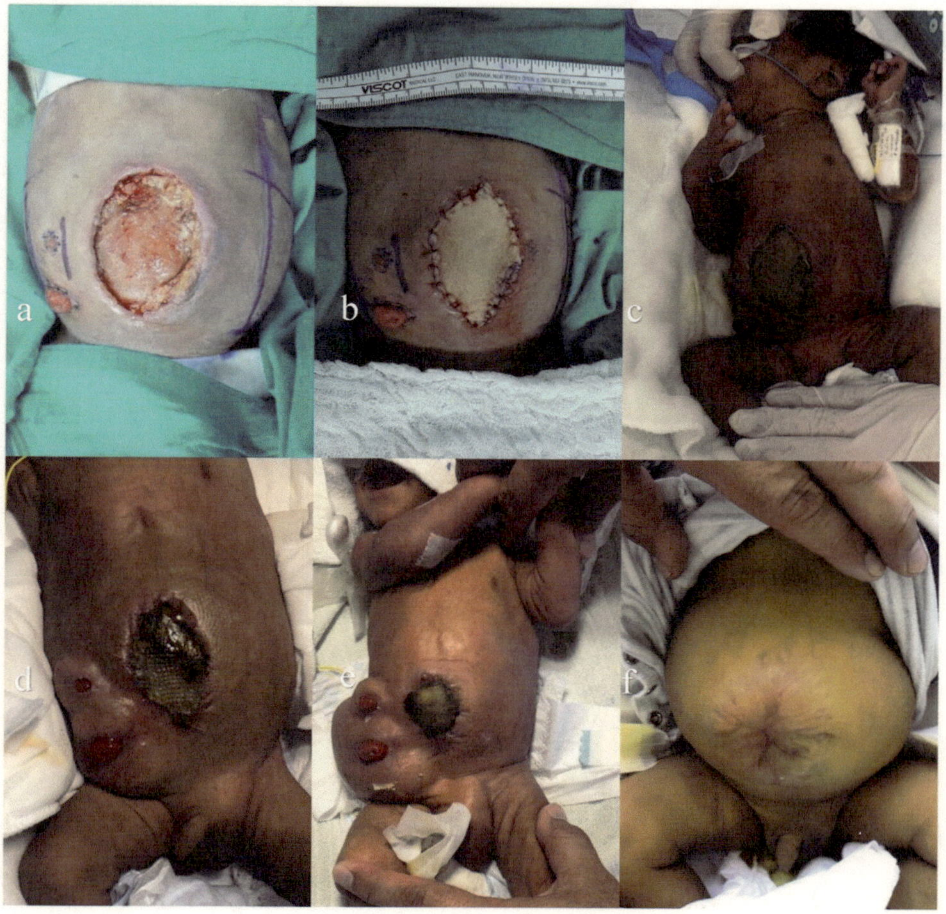

Figure 7.
30-week preterm infant. The patient evolves with necrotizing enterocolitis, requiring intestinal transit defunctionalization and evisceration on two occasions. a. Laparotomy contained. b. Immediate postoperative CTSA on open abdomen. c. Postoperative 21 days. d. Postoperative 35 days. e. Postoperative 60 days, protrusion of paraostomal hernia associated with Valsalva is observed, however the CTSA area shows continent, in addition to smaller size. f. Postoperative 90 days with healing by second intention, without intra-abdominal protrusion. Paraostomal hernias and transit reconstitution, associated with CTSA change performed on day 70.

5. Specifications

The therapeutic uses of CTSAs can be numerous. As we previously stated, we emphasize in our experience the diabetic foot, extensive and complex coverage deficits, contained laparotomies and post skin tumor resections, awaiting the biopsy results for an eventual margin enlargement and reconstruction (**Figures 6** and 7) [38–42]. CTSAs can cover bone, cartilage and tendon exposures, being a simple alternative for the management of complex wounds, becoming an intermediate coverage for some patients and definitive for others.

6. Conclusions

The distinctive characteristics of CTSAs (from living donor, full-thickness skin, and cryopreserved, therefore viable tissues) permits the obtention of a new type of coverage, which we have called intermediate coverage, easy to use, more economical than current alternatives and with numerous clinical indications.

Acknowledgements

The present study is an initial clinical experience, not a clinical trial, and was conducted under the supervision of the National Coordination of Organ and Tissue Procurement and Transplantation of the Chilean Ministry of Health.

Conflict of interest

The authors declare no conflict of interest.

Appendices and nomenclature

SA	Skin allograft
TSA	Total skin allograft
CTSA	Cryopreserved total skin allograft
NTB	National Tissue Bank
MRI	Magnetic Resonance Imaging

Author details

Marcelo Fonseca[1*], Aldo Cañete[2], Dino Ibaceta[1], Catalina Buchroithner[3], Florencia Disi[4] and Juan Olivares[5]

1 Department of Burns and Plastic Surgery, Dr. Ernesto Torres Galdames Hospital, Iquique, Chile

2 Organ and Tissue Procurement and Transplantation Unit, Dr. Ernesto Torres Galdames Hospital, Iquique, Chile

3 Departament of Dermatology, Dr. Ernesto Torres Galdames Hospital, Iquique, Chile

4 Department of Pathology, Dr. Ernesto Torres Galdames Hospital, Iquique, Chile

5 Department of Radiology, Dr. Ernesto Torres Galdames Hospital, Iquique, Chile

*Address all correspondence to: mfon777@hotmail.com

References

[1] Janis J, Kwon R, Attinger C. The new reconstructive ladder: modifications to the traditional model. Plast Reconstr Surg. 2011; 127, 205S-212S.

[2] Gottlieb LJ, Krieger LM. From the reconstructive ladder to the reconstructive elevator. Plast Reconstr Surg. 1994;93:1503– 1504.

[3] DiDomenico L, Emch K, Landsman A, Landsman A. A Prospective Comparison of Diabetic Foot Ulcers Treated With Either a Cryopreserved Skin Allograft or a Bioengineered Skin Substitute. Wounds, 2011; 23(7), 184-189.

[4] Leon-Villapalos J, Eldardiri M, Dziewulski P. The use of human deceased donor skin allograft in burn care. Cell and tissue banking, 2010; 11 (1), 99-104.

[5] Labuz D, Asch M, Buchmiller T. Use of Cadaveric Skin Graft for Staged Gastroschisis Repair in a Premature Infant. Neonatology, 2020; 117(5), 628-632.

[6] Gaucher S, Khaznadar Z, Gourevitch JC, Jarraya M. Skin donors and human skin allografts: evaluation of an 11-year practice and discard in a referral tissue bank. Cell and Tissue Banking, 2015; 17(1), 11–19.

[7] Dantzer E. Indicaciones de los sustitutos cutáneos y de los aloinjertos. EMC-Cirugía Plástica Reparadora y Estética, 2015; 23 (1): 1-14.

[8] Gaucher S, Jarraya M. Aloinjertos cutáneos en la cirugía del gran quemado. EMC-Cirugía Plástica Reparadora y Estética, 2009; 17(1): 1-10.pt

[9] Burd A, Chiu T. Allogenic skin in the treatment of burns. Clin Dermatol 2005; 23 (4): 376-387.

[10] Lazzeri D, Pantaloni M, Agostini T. Homografts and the Rejection Phenomenon: from burn care to organ transplantation. Plast Reconstr Surg 2010; 126(5), 1802-1803.

[11] Ben-Bassat H. Performance and safety of skin allografts. Clinics in dermatology, 2005; 23(4), 365-375.

[12] Dantzer E. Indicaciones de los sustitutos cutáneos y de los aloinjertos. EMC-Cirugía Plástica Reparadora y Estética, 2015; 23 (1): 1-14.

[13] Khoo TL, Halim AS, Saad AM, Dorai AA. The application of glycerol-preserved skin allograft in the treatment of burn injuries: an analysis based on indications. Burns 2010 36(6), 897-904.

[14] González F, Vera F, Alcayaga R, González F. Análisis crítico de la baja tasa de donación de órganos en Chile. Rev Med Chile 2020; 148: 242-251.

[15] Zúñiga-Fajuri A, Merino M, Urtubia *M. Una* mirada al origen, funcionamiento y desafíos del nuevo sistema de donación y trasplantes chileno. Rev Med Chile 2018; 146: 780-785.

[16] Zidan S, Eleowa S. Banking and use of glycerol preserved full-thickness skin allograft harvested from body contouring procedures. Burns, 2014 40 (4), 641-647.

[17] Friedland J, Maffi T. MOC-PS (SM) CME Article: Abdominoplasty. Plast Reconstr Surg 2008; 121(4), 1-11.

[18] Ministerio de Salud. Gobierno de Chile. Norma general técnica para el procuramiento, preservación e implante de tejidos. 2018.

[19] Morales-Olivera J, Plasencia J, Vázquez X. Cambios histológicos dérmicos tras pérdida masiva de peso y

su repercusión en la herida quirúrgica en abdominoplastia. Cirugía Plástica Ibero-Latinoamericana, 2019; 45(3), 275-283.

[20] Light D, Arvanitis G, Abramson D, Glasberg S. Effect of weight loss after bariatric surgery on skin and the extracellular matrix. Plast Reconstr Surg 2010; 125(1), 343-351.

[21] Martínez-Flores F, Sandoval-Zamora H, Machuca-Rodriguez C, Barrera-López A, García-Cavazos R, Madinaveitia-Villanueva J. Banco de piel y tejidos: un modelo operativo para la recuperación y preservación de aloinjertos de piel y tejidos. Cirugía y Cirujanos 2016; 84(1), 85-92.

[22] Pegg DE. Viability assays for preserved cells, tissues, and organs. Cryobiology 1989;26:212–31.

[23] Castagnoli C, Alotto D, Cambieri I, Casimiri R, Aluffi M, Stella M, et al. Evaluation of donor skin viability: fresh and cryopreserved skin using tetrazolioum salt assay. *Burns* 2003; **29**: 759-67.

[24] Gupta S. Optimal use of negative pressure wound therapy for skin grafts. International wound journal, 2012, vol. 9, p. 40-47.

[25] Stefanowska J, Zakowiecki D, Cal K. Magnetic resonance imaging of the skin. Journal of the European Academy of Dermatology and Venereology, 2010 24 (8), 875-880.

[26] Pomahac B, Garcia J, Lazar A, Tilney N, Orgill D. The skin allograft revisited: A potentially permanent wound coverage option in the critically ill patient. Plast Reconstr Surg 2009; 123 (6), 1755-1758.

[27] Knobloch K, Vogt P. Allograft skin as a permanent tissue repair: to mesh or not?. Plast Reconstr Surg 2010; 125(2), 750-751.

[28] Cuono C, Langdon R, Birchall N, Barttelbort S, McGuire J. Composite autologous-allogeneic skin replacement: development and clinical application. Plast Reconstr Surg 1987; 80(4), 626-637.

[29] Henn D, Chen K, Maan Z, Greco A, Moortgat Illouz S, Bonham C. et al. Cryopreserved human skin allografts promote angiogenesis and dermal regeneration in a murine model. International Wound Journal, 2020. 17 (4), 925-936.

[30] Burke J, Yannas I, Quinby W, Bondoc C, Jung W. Successful use of a physiologically aceptable artificial skin in the treatment of extensive burn injury. Ann Surg. 1981;194:413.

[31] Heimbach D, Luterman A, Burke J, Cram A, Herndon D, Hunt J et al. Artificial dermis for major burns. A multi-center randomized clinical trial. Ann Surg. 1988;208:313.

[32] Climov M, Bayer L, Moscoso A, Matsumine H, Orgill D. The role of dermal matrices in treating inflammatory and diabetic wounds. Plast Reconstr Surg 2016; 138(3S), 148S-157S.

[33] Monclús E, Perales A, Sanz E, Reola E, Agulló A. Utilización de matrices dérmicas en quemaduras. Cirugía Plástica Ibero-Latinoamericana, 2020;46, 39-46.

[34] Lee L, Porch J, Spenler W, Garner W. Integra in lower extremity reconstruction after burn injury. Plast Reconstr Surg. 2008;121:1256–1262.

[35] Schiavon M, Francescon M, Drigo D, Salloum G, Baraziol R, Tesei J. et al. The use of Integra dermal regeneration template versus flaps for reconstruction of full-thickness scalp defects involving the calvaria: A cost–benefit analysis. Aesthetic plastic surgery 2016; 40(6), 901-907.

[36] Roa R, Taladriz C. Uso actual de sustitutos dérmicos en cirugía reparadora. Revista chilena de cirugía, 2015, vol. 67, no 6, p. 647-652.

[37] Fonseca M, Cañete A, Ibaceta D, Gomez J, Santander M, Acuña P, Mandriaza L et al. Procuramiento y uso de aloinjertos cutáneos de piel total criopreservados obtenidos de pacientes sometidas a abdominoplastía. Rev. Cirugia. 2021;74(1). Disponible en: doi: 10.35687/s2452-4549%Y00%i1227 [Accessed 30 may. 2021].

[38] Bejarano P, Levi D, Nassiri M, Vincek V, Garcia M, Weppler D. et al. The pathology of full-thickness cadaver skin transplant for large abdominal defects: a proposed grading system for skin allograft acute rejection. The American journal of surgical pathology, 2004. 28(5), 670-675.

[39] Michielin O, Van Akkooi A, Ascierto P, Dummer R, Keilholz U. Cutaneous melanoma: ESMO Clinical Practice Guidelines for diagnosis, treatment and follow-up. Annals of Oncology 2019, 30(12), 1884-1901.

[40] Álvaro-Afonso F, García-Álvarez Y, Lázaro-Martínez J, Kakagia D, Papanas N. Advances in dermoepidermal skin substitutes for diabetic foot ulcers. Current vascular pharmacology, 2020 18(2), 182-192.

[41] Gordon A, Alfonso A, Nicholson J, Chiu E. Evidence for healing diabetic foot ulcers with biologic skin substitutes: a systematic review and meta-analysis. Annals of plastic surgery, 2019. 83(4S), S31-S44.

[42] DiDomenico L, Emch K, Landsman A, Landsman A. A Prospective Comparison of Diabetic Foot Ulcers Treated With Either a Cryopreserved Skin Allograft or a Bioengineered Skin Substitute. Wounds, 2011. 23(7), 184-189.